Living With Sarcoidosis
&
Other Chronic Health Conditions

Living With Sarcoidosis
&
Other Chronic Health Conditions

Patient Stories, Support Options,
Insurance Tips & A Physician Interview,
From A Patient's Perspective,
Reinforce The Fact... You're Not Alone!

Gilbert Barr, Jr.

iUniverse, Inc.
New York Lincoln Shanghai

Living With Sarcoidosis & Other Chronic Health Conditions

iUniverse, Inc.

For information address:
iUniverse, Inc.
2021 Pine Lake Road, Suite 100
Lincoln, NE 68512
www.iuniverse.com

ISBN: 0-595-32114-3

Printed in the United States of America

THIS BOOK IS DEDICATED TO ALL SARCOIDOSIS PATIENTS
BOTH PAST AND PRESENT
THEIR FAMILIES
AND
ALL CAREGIVERS

ALWAYS STAY POSITIVE!

Contents

FIRST THOUGHTS

I completed my first book, "*ME & SARCOIDOSIS—A LIFETIME PART-NERSHIP*" in April 2002, which gave a detailed account of my personal journey with my now partner for life...SARCOIDOSIS. Since that time I've traveled around the country speaking at various Sarcoidosis Awareness Events from New York to Los Angeles. In addition, I've had personal conversations and communicated via e-mail with sarcoidosis patients, sarcoidosis caregivers and doctors who support sarcoidosis patients/research, not only in this country but also around the world. I can honestly say that I've met some very courageous people who are dedicated to the mission of finding out everything we can about this still mysterious disease named sarcoidosis.

When it came time to write this book I wanted to take advantage of what I've learned from all of those courageous people about not only myself but also about their stories and how, although each sarcoidosis patient is unique (just like the individuals they are), we are all still the same and deal with the same issues in one way or another. People in general and with sarcoidosis share more in common than they share in differences. It's those similarities that we should concentrate on instead of the differences, which unfortunately seems to be what we do in America. Maybe one day we as a people will wake up and discover we really are one!

Hopefully, I've also learned a little about the publishing business. In reference to my first book I did everything myself, not wanting any outside influence or help regarding telling my story. As with all rookies I made several mistakes but as I've always been taught, no mistake is a mistake the first time as long as you take responsibility for it and learn from it. After all, if you don't make mistakes then you probably aren't doing anything. It's better to attempt something and make mistakes than not to attempt at all. That's a real tragedy!

One of my objectives for this book is to tell other patients' stories as well as mine and what I've experienced. This objective has been a very touching experience for me. As I hear some of the experiences others have endured dealing with sarcoidosis and their families, it makes me thankful for the many blessings I have. Staying positive is a major point I want to continually stress in my writings, communications and talks...It really does make a difference!

Each time I speak or e-mail a fellow patient or caregiver the similarities stand out, although each of our situations are slightly or dramatically different. Things like the misunderstanding by both the patient and those around them of what sarcoidosis is or how it affects a person depending on which organs are affected, the lack of concrete information available to them (although this is improving), lack of fellow patients to communicate with who understand what they experience, the seemingly misunderstanding or nonchalant attitude of a lot of medical professionals, employers and insurance companies (including Social Security) as to the seriousness of what sarcoidosis patients feel (if I only had a dime for every patient who has told me they were told they were crazy or their pain was mental before being diagnosed with sarcoidosis, including myself, then I would be a rich man!) and the overall mystery that still surrounds this disease, are just some of the things patients express as concerns. Every patient I've ever communicated with has expressed at least one of these concerns…Each and every time!

During the writing of this book I've also experienced two very personal and emotional events regarding patients who were going to be a part of this project. The first was the leader of a support group in New York City. When my first book came out she was an immediate supporter; in fact she gave me my first significant speaking engagement by inviting me to speak at her 2002 Annual Sarcoidosis Awareness Day and I was truly honored that she gave me that support. She was very soft spoken and confined to a wheel chair when I met her but she was so positive and full of life. I was to meet with her the last week in April 2003 to discuss her involvement with this project as I had a trip planned to New York City. The week before I was to leave we spent a long time talking on the phone about everything from our situations to how we wished others with sarcoidosis would stop the politics and start working together so we could hopefully make strides in the research and possible cure for sarcoidosis during our lifetime. Unfortunately she will never see that dream come true. Just a few days before I was to leave for New York City I received a call from a close associate in the support group; in fact we had tried to get him on the line with us the last time we spoke, a few nights prior. He informed me that she had passed away!

Anytime I hear a sarcoidosis patient passes away it brings a sense of reality to me that what we deal with is serious business. When you are trying to always stay positive and keep your head to the sky you (or at least I) tend to block that reality out. Even though I know of people who have passed away over the past years from complications due to sarcoidosis, some not even knowing they had sarcoidosis until after the fact, when it's someone you know and respect personally, plus was planning to meet in a couple of days, it really hits home. I will not only miss her, but even more so those who knew her on a daily basis will miss her. To be honest, even though I only spoke with her every couple of months, I truly cherished those conversations and valued the insight she provided to me. I will always be thankful I was able to know her and for the support she showed me!

Another patient, from the San Francisco Bay area, who also gave me immediate support when I released my first book, met personal tragedy in September 2003. She had agreed to provide her story and was actually going to be the main patient story featured in this book. I last spoke to her about a month prior as she was preparing for a trip to meet her father for the first time, a real dream for her. She had been feeling poorly lately but wanted to be involved by telling her story, so I was going to send her a detailed survey to fill out when she got back from her trip and we would go from there. As with my New York friend we had a nice long talk, as we always did. She was a true angel!

At the time I was also experiencing health and personal problems, plus it was going to be at least a couple of months before I was ready to start on her story, so I held off sending her the survey or calling. I wanted her to get some rest because she was the type of person who, when there is something to do regarding sarcoidosis, she is on it full blast and knowing her she was involved with something. In addition, I also knew she was having some health problems as well. She was supposed to have been a guest speaker at one of my workshops I was doing in the Los Angeles area in March 2003 but she was in the hospital at the time so I was not able to see her in person and because of that I knew she was still struggling. In fact, during that hospital visit they actually called in her family to give her their final goodbyes, but she wasn't ready to go yet.

Well, one September night in 2003 I got a call from a member of her support group, who I also knew personally, and she informed me my friend had passed away. Obviously this was a real personal blow to me and again hit home in regard to the seriousness of our disease. She touched a lot of lives in such a positive way. For me she was always supportive and would jump to my defense when anyone criticized my book, especially at the beginning when I had editing issues with the first couple of hundred or so copies that went out. Whenever I needed a positive lift, an e-mail between us would always do the trick. I still find it difficult to believe she is no longer with us although in spirit I feel she is looking down on us with her caring heart. The sarcoidosis community, her friends and most of all her family will truly miss her. I know I will!

Before I go any further I want to make something perfectly clear so that we have absolutely no misunderstandings in regard to my writings, speaking engagements or anything else you might hear from me. Whenever I speak I make sure this is the first thing that comes out of my mouth. **I am a patient!** I'm not a medical professional in any shape, form or size. I have no working experience or schooling as a Medical Physician, Psychiatrist, Nurse, Medical Assistant, Pharmacist, Lab Technician or any other field in the medical profession. I did, however, spend over 14 years with Electronic Data Systems supporting a national health care claims system for major corporations such as GM, Ford, Chrysler, K-Mart and others, underwritten by Blue Cross Blue Shield of Michigan and the other participating Blue Cross Blue Shield plans across the nation. From 1985 until 2000 I worked as a Data Center Manager responsible for the online and printing/ designing of forms, as a Project Manager going to various Blue Cross Blue Shield local plans to implement system and technical solutions, as a Financial Analyst responsible for the printing, mailing and accuracy of all financial documents and last as a Business Analyst responsible for implementing system changes and researching problems in regard to claim processing within the system. So I do have professional experience and an understanding of what goes on behind the scenes in regard to the processing of health care claims, at least up until the year 2000.

But first and foremost, I'm a patient. My experiences, opinions and perspectives are strictly from a patient's point of view. I always have the patient's best interest at heart. My writings come from my experiences as a patient, from my interactions and communications with other patients, my interactions and communications with those in the medical profession, including the insurance industry and government officials, from reading and researching information regarding sarcoidosis and last, but not least, from my personality, which based on my diverse background and the way I grew up allows me to see things in what I believe is reality. I believe in saying what's on my mind and taking nothing for granted or assume others see things the way I do. This is by no means saying I'm always right (just ask my wife about that) and if I'm wrong I'll be the first to admit it. However I do say what I believe based on my experiences and perspective. My point…When you hear me speak or read my writings always remember you are hearing or reading a patient's perspective. **Always!**

My ultimate objective for writing this book is as with the first book and all of my writings and speaking engagements is to bring awareness to sarcoidosis and the effect it has on patients…Period. This is my ultimate objective because if I'm successful with that objective then everything else for me personally will fall into place such as being able to support my family financially since people will buy my writings, strides will be made in patient support therefore benefiting me as a patient and hopefully strides will be made in obtaining a cure for sarcoidosis or maybe a better way of treating the disease without the many, many, many current drugs I take on a daily basis. So this is why I concentrate on bringing awareness to sarcoidosis and other chronic health conditions related to sarcoidosis from a patient's point of view. Who else can better describe how the disease affects your life than a fellow patient? I'm talking about coping with the every day struggles a sarcoidosis patient deals with, not treating the disease medically, we still need our doctors for that. But in regard to coping, no one knows better than an actual sarcoidosis patient! I don't care how much education you have or how many cases you have treated or studied, if you do not live with sarcoidosis on a daily basis and experience not only how it affects you but your family and those around you as well, then you really don't know, but then that's true with anything in life, isn't it?

Sarcoidosis?...

So what is sarcoidosis? That's a million dollar question if I ever heard one! When I'm asked that question this is my general answer. "Sarcoidosis is an autoimmune disease that can affect any organ or gland in the body including the eyes, skin and spine in the form of granulomas, which are basically lumps that develop in organs or glands when cells from the immune system clump together. Sarcoidosis can affect anyone regardless of race, sex, age, living or working environments, financial status, political affiliations, sense of humor or any other factor you can think of. There is currently no known origin for the disease although several theories exist such as something in the environment causes the immune system to overreact, possibly some type of bacteria, genetic or maybe a combination of some type...We just do not know for sure but strides are being made. There are no "standard" tests that are run to detect sarcoidosis nor is there a legal definition or category that truly defines the disease and the many off spins that can occur from sarcoidosis. Last, but not least, there is currently no cure for sarcoidosis! Sarcoidosis is a perfect example of something that shows absolutely no prejudice! Any organ/gland...Any one...At any time! No known cause and no known cure!"

This is why there is such a need for continued research and studies, but we must be careful in both of these aspects so that we take full advantage of any opportunities we come across to learn more about sarcoidosis. We can't let personal agendas and a lack of participants from all walks of life interfere with true progress in our journey for knowledge and understanding regarding sarcoidosis.

Research, for example, must be rid of politics and unethical behavior. Unfortunately, like anything in life when funding is at stake, there will be shady doings, even in such an important field as medical research. This is just a fact of life so let's face it and address it head on. We as sarcoidosis patients and as a society have too much at stake for such nonsense. The same holds true for studies as the results of a study can make or break a corporation based on the findings. Those who can profit from a specific finding should not be involved in the study. Look at the fine print of a lot of the drug studies and see who provided funding. Is it a coincidence that the results usually come out in the favor of those contributors? You be the judge.

Independent studies should be the norm and research should be conducted with an open mind. We have too many brilliant medical professionals and scientists to not understand more about sarcoidosis and the medical effects it has on people's lives. We should not have to wait for misdiagnosis or a biopsy to finally diagnose a patient with sarcoidosis, sometimes taking months and even years. We should not have to wait for patients to constantly die in order to take this seriously. With modern technology we should and could know more!

In addition we need our elected officials to start looking at legislation to help sarcoidosis patients and fund sarcoidosis research. I understand that sarcoidosis research is not on the top of the critical list for politicians to get elected, but health care is and the caring of sarcoidosis patients is part of our health care issues in America. As of the beginning of 2004 there isn't a substantial legal definition nor category for sarcoidosis, as patients are constantly denied needed benefits from Social Security, insurance companies and employers...This has to change as well! As a sarcoidosis patient I feel the effect of these situations but the reality is we are all affected. Chronic health conditions affect everyone in one way or another, especially with the number of uninsured Americans in today's world.

It's time to get serious about sarcoidosis awareness so please read this book with an open mind and practice what Funk Legend George Clinton has been chanting since the 1970s and title of a Funkadelic song…"**THINK! It Ain't Illegal Yet!**"

1

ME & SARCOIDOSIS

✦

A Continuing Saga

Since the release of "*ME & SARCOIDOSIS—A LIFETIME PARTNER-SHIP*" I've learned so much about myself, along with the effect living with sarcoidosis has on my life, from both a personal and medical perspective. I've been blessed to have the opportunity to meet so many others who also have this mysterious disease and have learned so much from them as well. Before the release of my story I could easily count the number of people I knew with sarcoidosis on one hand, now I would need pages. Each time I hear a new story, have the opportunity to speak to a new patient, receive an e-mail from someone with sarcoidosis or communicate with someone who has a person close to them with the disease, it touches my heart in a very unique and special way. Although our cases are different in many ways, based on several factors, the main being which organs are affected with the sarcoidosis granulomas or the secondary conditions we have developed, there are always common experiences and feelings we share…Each and every time. This is why I continue to tell my very personal story!

I was born in February 1958. Due to a complicated birth, I grew up an only child in North Florida (Perry and Tallahassee). My pre-sarcoidosis life was filled with athletic activities and I was always full of energy. My father was a basketball coach and, as it would turn out, I was an athlete, primarily basketball—however, I also played baseball, tennis, swam and any other activity that was going on in the neighborhood. Aside from a wet sinus problem, I was in great physical health and was very seldom sick with anything, basically an average kid, if there is such a thing.

I moved to Detroit, Michigan in October 1985 (I was 27 years old) to work for Electronic Data Systems (EDS). Upon arriving in Detroit, I immediately started to have a change in my sinus problem, going from wet mucus to hard

1

mucus. This caused me several problems, such as trouble breathing and being short of breath. However, the most painful result of this new sinus problem was migraine headaches.

My migraines were very specific each and every time. They would start anywhere from 30 minutes to a couple of hours after I would unsuccessfully attempt to blow my nose, usually the left side. They would only occur in the left corner of my right eye and would feel as if someone was touching, then holding down on a nerve, similar to a dentist before your exposed tooth nerve is numb. Then instantly, and I mean within seconds, not gradually over time, they would just stop...Completely. This would truly amaze me and I could not understand it, but the relief was so welcomed.

When I would have the migraines I would hurt so badly that I would, at times, literally hit myself in other parts of my body, so I could feel pain somewhere else. I would usually vomit mucus, then blood, and would be soaking wet with sweat, but yet my body would be cold to the touch. The migraines started on a regular basis around the end of 1986 and beginning of 1987 and the vomiting of mucus and blood from my nose became a daily occurrence around 1988. These migraine headaches were the most painful situation I've ever experienced to this day and except for catching a buzz to ease the mental burden for a brief time, no medications I was ever given even put a dent in the pain!

As the migraines started occurring more frequently, and by mid-1988 were occurring pretty much on a daily basis, other symptoms started to pop up as well. I started to become thirsty on a frequent basis and the thirst was nothing I had experienced before. It could best be described as intense, because if I didn't get something to drink I would literally start to shake, similar to a junkie going cold turkey, as my throat and mouth would become extremely dry. As a result of the increased liquid intake, I started to urinate more frequently as well. Again, it was like nothing I had experienced before. My urine was completely clear and you could forget about holding it, as I normally could in the past. It would actually be very painful. Around this time my nights started to consist of me waking up every couple of hours to get something to drink then urinate before going back to sleep for another couple of hours. In the morning I would normally vomit before starting my day. This went on every single night for years!

My appetite started to decrease and, as a result, I started to drop weight at a fairly rapid rate. My meals would basically consist of a few bites and a lot to drink. I even started a diet of Carnation Instant Breakfast and baby juice, since it was easier to drink than eat. Still, I would usually vomit most of it up after a short time.

With the combination of not being able to eat, losing weight, and the fact I couldn't sleep more than a couple of hours at a time, my energy levels and strength dramatically decreased, to the point that it altered my everyday life. Playing basketball became an almost impossible struggle, as after a couple of games I would get extremely hot, but yet I was not sweating and my body was physically cold to the touch. Then that "tingling" feeling would hit me, as my throat and mouth became extremely dry. You know that feeling when you know you don't have much time left before something is coming up. Sure enough, the next thing I knew I was in the restroom vomiting mucus and blood from my nose. That would be the end of my game for that day. Finally, around the beginning of 1990 I just gave up. That forced decision not only hurt me physically, as now with the lack of exercise I just got weaker and weaker, but for me it was the mental aspect that hurt the most, since basketball was more than just a game to me. Sometimes the mental torment is worse than any physical pain you might experience and a lot harder to deal with. My life was starting to change in a downward spiral that was starting to scare me.

My skin started to change and gave me two specific problems. The first was my face started to become two-toned. I would have dark spots all over my face in no particular pattern, as the rest of my skin was turning a ghostly white. I was real scary looking! In addition, I started to develop tiny red blisters on my arms, usually my left one which was exposed to the sun when I drove, that itched awfully. I was told it was skin poisoning from being exposed to the sun, which didn't make sense to me since I grew up in Florida and had never even used sunscreen nor ever had any problems with sunburn and—remember, my favorite pastime was playing basketball on the playgrounds in the hot Florida weather. Now all of a sudden I can't even drive without getting "skin poisoning"? Something just didn't make sense with that explanation.

To add to my new look, my eyes were starting to bulge out as if they were about to pop out of my face and the bones in my neck or Adams Apple would be best described as real skeleton looking. It got to where I scared myself, or at least had to look twice when I walked past a mirror to make sure it was still me I was looking at. Again, the mental aspect of my changed appearance, combined with the lack of physical activity, was starting to get the best of me.

I kept telling myself to stay strong and dug deep inside my soul, but I knew I was starting to weaken mentally as well as physically. All I could do was keep my strong faith in God for strength and guidance. God is my inner strength and I knew He or She would take care of me, but as a human being in times of pain and uncertainty...Although I never doubted, I still worried.

Other problems started to occur as well, such as severe muscle cramps, although my muscles were actually shrinking, my feet and heels were becoming hard and cracked, I would cough when I would talk, especially when on the phone, not being able to complete a couple of sentences at a time and I was having shortness of breath more frequently. Then there was still the everyday routine of vomiting mucus and blood along with constant slow nosebleeds at all times of the day and night. I would constantly wake up to blood spots on my pillowcase.

Then to top it off, I started to develop male hormone problems, such as my facial hair started to thin out, my breasts started to grow, my erections were not as hard as they should be, although hard enough to perform intercourse most times, I was not producing any semen and my testicles were shrinking. I had just met my future wife about this time, which added to the frustration of my new problems. The positive factor was she was now in my life. I knew she was my soul mate from the first time our eyes met! It just took courage and help from her for us to get together. It's hard enough to develop and maintain an honest strong relationship, whether it's a friendship or romantic partnership, but when you have health problems and are sick most of the time it's even more challenging. Your outlook on interfacing with others is less than desirable, to put it mildly. It takes a lot of strength to just go out in public and deal with other people, whether it's on a personal or business level. Even interfacing with strangers in small talk situations is not something you look forward to. So I must admit, I was blessed by God to have my soul mate come into my life at this time. It made all the positive difference in the world because by this time I was a mess, both physically and mentally!

Since the start of my problems in 1986 until 1990, I saw seven different Internal or Family Practice Physicians, based on which ones my insurance policy allowed me to see at the time. Each one would put me through the same routine consisting of a complete physical, blood tests, chest X-ray and test my sugar levels for diabetes. Then each one had the same result for all of the symptoms I was experiencing…I had bad sinus problems. The sinus problems were causing a chain reaction within my body and when the weather changed I should be okay, although it had been years now and the weather had changed several times, but until then I could take pain pills for my migraines. This made absolutely no sense to me! All it did was add to the mental frustration, not to mention the obvious fact my physical health was deteriorating on a daily basis. If not for the guidance of God, my newfound soul mate and my internal mental strength, I would have gone crazy. In fact, I know several patients who were told they were crazy and were referred for psychiatric help before being diagnosed with sarcoidosis.

Although not told this directly, it was hinted and mentioned that a lot of my symptoms were probably just in my head.

Getting sicker by the day and not having anywhere to turn for help is an awful feeling! Sarcoidosis patients especially understand this pre-diagnosis feeling because it seems a lot of us have been misdiagnosed for a prolonged period of time, which in turn causes other chronic health conditions to develop. We must have standard medical tests, other than biopsies to look for sarcoidosis, instead of just waiting for other diagnoses to be wrong. These tests should not only be conducted regularly by our primary physicians but also be available at health fairs and free clinics, since unfortunately in today's environment there are a lot of people without health care insurance. They deserve to be tested for sarcoidosis as well. After all, in the end it will be the taxpayers who support their care, so why not try a "prevent mode" approach? We must understand that this crisis, and the health care insurance situation in America is a crisis, affects us all. It's not just the poor folks who are now without insurance coverage these days. Look at who is unemployed. Regardless of who you are, I bet you don't have to look very far to find someone you know without coverage.

As the majority of the people in this country who rely on their insurance for their health care options, along with the fact I was new to town, my choices were pretty much a needle in a haystack or based on someone I met for a personal referral. However, I didn't know anyone with all of the symptoms I was experiencing, therefore my referral pool was shallow. Then, of course, my insurance had to allow me to see their doctors anyway. It amazed me after the release of *"ME & SARCOIDOSIS—A LIFETIME PARTNERSHIP"* when I would hear people with money, clout or political connections, or live in a wealthy community tell me that they never had any problems with their medical professionals and I was just being negative because the medical community doesn't treat people like that. It was my attitude that caused me to experience my problems. There were only a few of those comments and they always kept their names anonymous (real brave people!), although other factors gave away things about them, but just the fact people think like that amazed me and enforced the reason we have these problems, especially when treating sarcoidosis or any other autoimmune disease that remains so mysterious. Trust me, it happened to me and as I've spoken with many patients since, it happens more often than you think. I'm just one straw in the haystack that's been forming for years! So don't get mad at me for telling my story.

I want to make something perfectly clear before we move on…I'm not negative with regard to the medical profession. I have many qualified doctors and deal with others in the medical profession with positive results. I just tell my story and experiences as they happened. What happened, happened, and I can't change those facts, although I wish I could. My quality of life sure would be a lot better! I understand it's hard to be a doctor, as the human body is a complicated natural machine. As I just said, over the years I've had many superb doctors whom I credit with keeping me alive and as healthy as possible. After all, without them I could be a lot worse. As patients we need our doctors to survive. My point and all I asked regarding the medical professionals who I dealt with at that time in my life, and for that matter the medical professionals I deal with now, was if they didn't know then ask for help. Not a single one of them sent me to any kind of specialist. Instead, each one rushed me in and out of their office with a result that just didn't make sense. Think about this for a second. I saw several of these doctors for over a year and their diagnosis for **all** my symptoms was sinus problems. Their solution was pain pills and when the seasons changed I would be okay. The seasons changed several times while I was under their care and the only changes I experienced were negative. But yet their solution remained the same, except to hint that some of my symptoms might be mental. If just one of them asked for help then I wouldn't be writing this book today because my sarcoidosis might not have spread throughout my body causing me to have many permanent secondary chronic health conditions…For life! That's what makes me bitter every time I think about it or hear others tell me their stories that are too similar for comfort to mine! Reality is reality!

At this point I didn't know what to do, except continue to pray to God for guidance. My life was changing all around me and except for my soul mate, new stepdaughter and still being alive, the changes were all negative and getting worse each and every day. My interaction with other people, on both a professional and personal level, was a struggle, even those I loved and only had my best interest in mind. It's hard to be around others when you are sick and no one can tell you why or help you. It's a mental burden that you carry with you around the clock and talking about it with others is very difficult to do, even to those extremely close to you who want to do everything they can to help you. I stopped exercising completely because I would just vomit and was too weak to put forth much effort. I was missing a lot of work. I was falling asleep at the drop of a hat. I even fell asleep standing up leaning against a wall a few times. Of course the sleep was never that deep necessary sleep our bodies need because I would always wake up in a couple of hours for my now normal routine of urinating and possibly vomiting then drinking some type of fluid before going back to sleep until the next time, which like clockwork would occur within two hours…Every single day and night for years! In other words, I was at my mental breaking point and I prayed God would show me a sign!

The Sign…

Fortunately, as always when I reach my physical and mental breaking point, God came through. One day in mid-1990 I went to the mailbox and in my junk mail was a coupon for a free consultation with a Chiropractor just down the street. For some unknown reason (actually it was God subliminally communicating with me), I didn't throw the coupon away but instead put it on my table, even though I knew my insurance didn't cover Chiropractor visits. After my next daily migraine, I decided to put aside my fear of being cracked, as I can't even stand to hear someone pop their knuckles, and the fact my insurance didn't cover the service, and took him up on the free visit.

After some brief/detailed conversation and an X-ray, he determined what was causing my migraines. It seems the top bone in my cervical vertebrae was just slightly off center. As a result when my sinus cavity would fill with hard mucus it caused the off-center bone to press against a nerve that affected the left corner of my right eye. When the mucus would finally drain then the bone released contact, which in turn gave immediate relief, as the nerve was no longer having pressure applied to it. Finally, an explanation that actually made logical sense! To add to this scenario, since my mother had a hard time giving birth to me, the bone was probably off center my entire life, but it wasn't until my sinus changed from wet to hard mucus that it caused the migraines. Just hearing a medical professional, although the conservative medical community didn't consider Chiropractors on their level at this time, give me a logical explanation gave me major mental relief and more importantly…Hope! My prayers had been answered!

There was still one minor problem…My insurance didn't cover the service. So as I recommend everyone do, I discussed cost openly and upfront. Just because it's a doctor and involves your health is not a reason for you not to be concerned about cost the way you are about other things in your life in which you spend your money for. If a doctor is in the business of truly helping their patients then they will work with you if you are honest and upfront about your financial state. If your doctor isn't willing to listen to your concern and attempt to make what is needed for you a reality from a financial standpoint, then he or she might not be the doctor for you anyway. Get a second opinion…Fast! It's not only your health at stake but your money as well. After all, both factors contribute to your overall quality of life.

His normal fee to those with insurance was $88 per session. For me he would charge $44 per session. This was still a little out of my range since we were looking at twice a week sessions for a total of six weeks, so he suggested I talk to his office manager to see if we could work anything additional out. The final deal came to $22 per session, cash. So by me being upfront about my financial situation my cost went from a total of $1,056 to $264, for a difference of $792 for my treatment program. Not only did it pay off financially, but also from a health standpoint it was a major success.

My treatment plan consisted of twice a week sessions for six weeks in which my neck and spine were adjusted, along with my sinus cavities massaged. The treatments used no drugs, therefore I had no related side effects, only muscle soreness from the adjustments, similar to a hard workout. As a result of the treatment my migraines went away on schedule and to this day have never returned.

Please always keep your options and mind open in regard to your health, or anything in your life for that matter. If I hadn't kept the free coupon from my junk mail, then faced my fear of being popped or adjusted, then I might have never gotten rid of the most painful experience I've ever encountered. This situation also paved the path for future success to come.

The other thing I did, which again I recommend everyone do regardless of what profession or activity you are dealing with, is when you find someone who you have had success with but yet you still need additional help…Ask for a referral to someone they work with or are associated with. This holds true for all professions and activities, whether it be someone who did great work on your home or works on your car, or maybe someone who is even good in sports and you need another player for your team, but especially in the medical profession where there are so many specialties, and you usually need several specialists to get to the bottom of a serious medical condition. The reason I stress this is because the fact is that successful people surround themselves with other successful people…Period. In the past my choice of doctors had been based strictly on who my insurance policy allowed me to see then who was closer to my home or office. Now that I finally had success, I wasn't about to let this opportunity slip away! The Chiropractor referred me to a doctor he worked with directly and was his Personal Physician. I immediately made an appointment.

I spent the next few months with the referred doctor trying to find what was causing all of my other health problems. He ran me through the same routines, only he added a few new twists to the testing process with MRIs and CAT scans plus tried a few new medications such as cortisone six-packs. We developed a good relationship over the next couple of months and spoke honestly to each other about what was going on with me physically and mentally. In February 1991 he called me into his office for a serious talk.

He started by telling me he had an idea as to what was causing my problems and it wasn't sinus problems, but instead there was something wrong with my pituitary gland…He just didn't know what or, for that matter, what to do about it. However, he was certain that if nothing was done fast then in two to three weeks I would fall asleep and never wake up. He had no doubt that within a month I would be dead! As deep as that conversation was it didn't take me by surprise, after all, I had been getting worse over the past few years and especially over the past few months and the reality is you can only get so bad. But more than anything I appreciated his honesty so my response was, "So what are we going to do about it?"

He told me he wanted to send me to an Endocrinologist for additional tests and would call ahead to explain the situation so I didn't have to wait due to me being a new patient. For the first time during this long ordeal I was experiencing a real professional who admitted he didn't know and was asking for help. All I've ever asked from any medical professional is that if you don't know, please ask for help instead of, for whatever reasons, not wanting others to think you don't understand. The human body is a complicated natural machine, but more importantly, you are dealing with someone's life and your lack of decision could have permanent dramatic effects. Just imagine how my life might be if only one of the previous seven doctors since 1986 had just asked for a second opinion when their first opinion obviously wasn't working. Oh well, I can't do anything about the past except tell my story to anyone who will listen.

After one more round of tests with the Endocrinologist, as he wanted to start his own records, it was exactly as he had expected. He told me I had a disease called sarcoidosis. Although there was no known origin for the disease he could tell me that it's an autoimmune disease that causes a buildup of inflammatory cells in your tissue. The inflammatory cells form a pattern of inflammation known as granulomas, which are basically lumps that develop when cells from the immune system overreact for some unknown reason. In my case, the sarcoidosis started in my lungs then spread to my liver and lymph nodes. Then it moved to my brain where it started building up on my pituitary gland. In layman terms, once it hit my pituitary gland, it was killing the cells or functions of the pituitary gland it came in contact with, therefore causing the pituitary gland not to produce the appropriate steroids or hormones my body needed to survive.

He told me there was no cure for sarcoidosis but we could treat it successfully. The treatment would consist of replacement medications to give me what my body should be producing on its own, along with an initial large dose of prednisone to put the sarcoidosis in remission. With consistent monitoring we could keep the sarcoidosis under control and although I wouldn't live the same life as I did prior to 1986, it was not the end of the world and I could still live a fulfilling and productive but yet different life. It was now April 1991 and I had a new partner for life...Sarcoidosis!

Time To Move On...

The initial physical results from the location of sarcoidosis consisted of several now permanent secondary conditions. They included not being able to get the proper amount of air out of my lungs and shortness of breath. Although the majority of sarcoidosis cases affect the lungs (but please keep in mind sarcoidosis can affect any organ or gland in your body including the eyes, skin and spine) it is not just a lung disease. These were really the only specific lung problems I had, as of now.

Other conditions included an overactive immune system, hypopituitarism, hypothyroidism, insufficient testosterone levels, insufficient potassium levels, diabetes insipidus (water diabetes), weak bones and muscles, an overall insufficient endocrine system and chronic fatigue.

To combat these health conditions I would start by taking prednisone on a daily basis several times a day. The prednisone had a multitude of purposes, the first being at a high dose to put the sarcoidosis in remission, which was successful in about six to eight weeks. Prednisone would become my life saving drug, as it does so much good for me, even though there are many side effects and a lot of patients have problems dealing with both the physical and mental side effects. Some of the side effects I experienced, and still do, include weight gain, puffy or round face, appetite increase, mood swings and muscle cramps, along with swollen legs. Fortunately, I don't have any problems taking prednisone, other than the side effects mentioned. My mother, for example, breaks out badly, even on a small dose. I know patients for various reasons that flat out refuse to take the drug, especially those with joint problems as prednisone can have a negative effect on the affected joints. A fairly large number of hip replacements with sarcoidosis patients are reported with prednisone being the main cause for the problem. Unfortunately, for those sarcoidosis patients, prednisone is one of the most popular drugs used to control sarcoidosis. With increased research other alternate drugs and treatments are being discovered. But for me, prednisone does the trick and one positive is it's cheap.

A hint…If you have a high co-pay on your prescription coverage and you are limited to a one month supply, see what it would cost you to pay for your prescription out of pocket and have your doctor write a high quantity. A lot of times you will come out cheaper once you do the math. Another tip to get over the one-month clause is to have your doctor write a specific quantity then for the dosage instructions write "Take As Directed". This helps me because if I have any changes such as weight gain, additional stress in my life, any type of cold or infection or any other type of health or emotional change, then I have to take additional prednisone. Therefore, when I would go to get my prescription refilled, it would be denied, because my one-month timeframe was not up…A real hassle, especially since I need prednisone to survive. This way I don't have that problem. One last thing regarding prednisone, you can't just stop taking it! This will be very dangerous for you. You must slowly reduce your intake over a period of time. Please consult with your medical professional when you are in this situation. Do not mess around with prednisone!

For my hypothyroidism I take synthroid. This was the reason I had such symptoms as holding heat inside my body, my facial spotting, my neck and eyes bulging and a lack of energy. Synthroid doesn't give me many side effects although I do experience severe muscle cramps, which is a side effect of synthroid. However, muscle cramps are a side effect of almost all of the medications I take along with a result of certain levels such as testosterone or potassium being low. Who knows what each individual muscle cramp is caused from since I have them on a daily basis? We quit trying to figure that out years ago! There has been a lot of bad press about synthroid over the years, such as inconsistencies and fights with the FDA. But from my perspective and my Endocrinologist, it works just fine for me.

The last daily medication I was to take was DDAVP, which is a nasal spray for my diabetes insipidus. Diabetes insipidus is a rare form of diabetes (although it's not technically categorized as a diabetic disease) that causes extreme thirst and urination like no thirst or sensation you have ever experienced. My diabetes insipidus is caused because of the fact that my body no longer produces the hormone vasopressin (anti-diuretic hormone [ADH]), which is produced in the posterior lobe of the pituitary gland due to sarcoidosis affecting that portion of my brain. The lack of effect of this hormone on the kidney causes excretion of excessive quantities of very diluted, but otherwise normal, urine. Most people only think of the kidneys in regard to urination problems but the brain, or more specifically the pituitary gland, also should be considered. This is why the feelings I experienced regarding my thirst and having to urinate was so intense and like nothing I had felt before. Fortunately for me, DDAVP had just recently been dis-covered; otherwise I would have required four daily injections into my kidneys. I guess my luck was changing for the better after all because to this day needles are a major weakness of mine.

Speaking of needles, for my insufficient testosterone levels, which caused my male hormone problems, weak bones and muscles along with mood swings and lack of energy, I was going to have to get a bi-weekly muscle injection of depo-testosterone. Since giving the injection myself was out of the question, I go to the doctor's office and have a nurse administer the injection for me. I've gone every other week since April 1991. It's a hassle but well worth the results.

There are a couple of other ways to take testosterone, and I've tried both with-out positive results. The first is by way of a daily patch. I personally hated wearing a patch, as it was uncomfortable and a hassle, to me personally. The next and what I believe would be the best way, is with a daily gel that you apply each morning. After a couple of hours you can do anything, including get into water, something you couldn't do with a patch on. It was a perfect solution, however my body would never accept the medication for some unknown reason. I tried it twice at the highest dosages we could go, in fact the dosage was so high my insur-ance would only cover half of the prescription a month, but my body just kept rejecting it. I'm the only patient my Endocrinologist has seen whose body reacts that way to the gel. Just my luck!

Life Goes On As Changes Continue…

Since my first diagnosis for sarcoidosis in 1991, I've developed several additional permanent secondary conditions. Hypertension is one of those conditions that I developed a few years after my diagnosis. I currently take medication twice daily and the dosage has been increased several times over the years. Another condition is severe acid reflux due to the fact that my esophagus doesn't open all of the way causing stomach acid or food to back up. Since the esophagus has no protective mucosal layer the acid causes severe pain just behind the sternum (breastbone) and seems to come from the heart. This is where the term "heartburn" comes from and in my case it is extremely painful when it occurs. I've actually known two grown men who went to the emergency room thinking they were having a heart attack when it was only (and I write that lightly) acid reflux. I take a daily tablet for that condition as well.

In 2000 I developed sleep apnea and must now sleep with a Continuous Posi-tive Airway Pressure machine, or better known as a CPAP machine, on a nightly basis. Sleep apnea is very common (as common as adult diabetes) and affects more than 12 million Americans (according to the National Institutes of Health in 2003). Common risk factors include being male, overweight, and over the age of 40. But, like sarcoidosis, sleep apnea can strike anyone at any age, even children and should not be stereotyped into only one group of people. Everyone is at risk! Also, like sarcoidosis, because of the lack of awareness by the public and healthcare professionals, the vast majority of patients remain undiagnosed and therefore untreated, despite the fact that this serious disorder can have significant consequences.

Untreated, sleep apnea can cause high blood pressure and other cardiovascular disease, memory problems, weight gain, impotency, relationship problems (if you sleep with someone who snores you understand) and headaches. Moreover, untreated sleep apnea may be responsible for job impairment and motor vehicle crashes since your body must have sleep in order to function properly. Fortunately, sleep apnea can be diagnosed and treated, as mine was. It took a while to get used to sleeping with the CPAP machine, which is basically a mask over your nose with a tube going to a small machine that continuously keeps air flowing into your nose, but now I wouldn't go anywhere without it.

Around this time, after spending almost a year with no feeling in my feet, I was diagnosed with bad nerve endings as a result of diabetes mellitus (sugar diabetes). I take medication three times a day to help restore and maintain my nerve endings. For my diabetes mellitus I started by controlling it via my diet and walking, however that has changed. As of now I take medication via a tablet at each meal. In addition I now check my blood sugar levels four times daily and give the readings to my Endocrinologist every two weeks when I get my depo-testosterone injection. Like I wrote earlier I'm scared of needles, but I should realize that a few daily pokes in the finger is better than having to inject myself with insulin several times a day. However, as of late, my sugar readings are climbing and climbing on a regular basis, as they now average around 200 to 225 before meals and over 300, and at times in the 400 ranges, when tested two hours after meals. Per my Endocrinologist the ranges should average 140 before meals and 170 after meals, so as you can see they are out of range on a daily basis. In fact first thing in the morning they should average 100 but they are always over 180 and lately over 200. I don't know how much longer a tablet is going to be sufficient, as my Endocrinologist told me insulin was definitely in my future and I had to try and walk at least 20 minutes every day. My educated guess is that before this book is published I'll be on insulin.

During my last appointment I told my Endocrinologist that my main goal was to stay off insulin, in which he replied sternly, "No, your goal is to live as long as you can and stay as healthy as you can, regardless of what it takes!" Okay, better put. I'm just going to have to dig down deep in my soul and ask for help from God to get over my fear of needles. To be honest, I do feel pretty lousy most of the time these days. It's just very frustrating to continue to develop additional conditions and then they get worse but yet according to the experts all I'm supposed to be suffering from with sarcoidosis is shortness of breath, aching joints and maybe a little fatigue. I wish whoever wrote those definitions could live in my body for a day!

Other somewhat minor, but constant problems I experience, include vision and dental. Trust me, those are two areas of your body that you better not play around with, so maybe I shouldn't have used the words "somewhat minor" to describe the problems. From a vision standpoint I have several factors as to why I must get my eyes checked at least once a year. Having sarcoidosis, taking prednisone for a prolonged period of time, and having diabetes are red flags for vision problems. Oh yeah, if you must wear glasses, wear them! As far as taking care of your dental needs, this can be more important than you think. Again, because of such factors as sarcoidosis and diabetes (both insipidus and mellitus), I have a high risk of dental problems. Your teeth, or more specifically decay in your teeth, will cause you problems throughout your body and you might not even realize the core of the problem. When the bacterium gets in your bloodstream it can travel all over your body. In my case, with sarcoidosis and an overactive immune system, unless I know to take additional prednisone I can develop other problems. Then with diabetes mellitus when an infection or foreign bacterium enters your body it will find the weakest part of the body to attack. As for the diabetes insipidus, since I don't produce the proper amount of saliva, my teeth are subject to decay and becoming brittle. Take care of your dental needs! With today's technology it isn't as bad as you might think. Remember keep an open mind and dig deep inside yourself to overcome any fears you might have because your health is at stake. Remember my Chiropractor situation?

One hint to mention, and although it might sound simple or crazy to you, is pay attention to your body scents. If you have bad breath then that could be a sign of tooth decay. If you seem to produce a strong or bad body odor and you keep yourself clean and use good body hygiene, then that could be a sign something in your body is not working correctly. This is a situation, although hard to address, that needs to be addressed by your caregiver or those around you. Your body will try and give you signs when things aren't working correctly…Learn to read your own signs honestly then get help as soon as possible. Never be embarrassed to tell your doctor about anything you think is unusual. It's your health at stake!

Next is my high cholesterol, that I currently take medication to control. I know I should be watching my diet more to control the high cholesterol and my diabetes mellitus but I must confess this is hard for me. There were two things that I couldn't do before my diagnosis that I now cherish every single time I do either. The first is making love to my wife. The other is eating. Plus with my diabetes mellitus getting worse, which can make you hungry and my intake of prednisone, which makes you have the munchies all the time, controlling my diet is a real challenge but one I must be aware of at all times. Of course exercising, such as walking daily, would also help. To top it off I also suffer from hemorrhoids, but like most people I just deal with them for now.

One last thing (at least for now) to add to my conditions is I have developed an irregular heartbeat, which I've found is somewhat common among sarcoidosis patients. I've had several stress tests (which I was unable to complete due to other health issues) and we are still not sure of the actual cause. It was determined that the sarcoidosis has not spread to my heart, however, I have several factors other than sarcoidosis such as diabetes, high cholesterol, prolonged intake of prednisone and who knows what else, that could be causing the irregular heartbeat. My heart specialist named seven other factors. So for now I take a baby aspirin daily and will have a follow-up every five months or so to monitor the situation. I'm also in a heart safety program via my HMO, the same with my diabetes mellitus. This is one good thing my HMO does, as it provided tips on living with these conditions at no additional charge. Still, I don't feel too comfortable with this wait and see process with my heart, but what can I do? So in the meantime I try to stay calm, as much as possible, and put my faith in God. Life is too precious to waste getting upset about minor everyday things that you can't really do anything about anyway. As the saying goes, "Don't sweat the small stuff!"

Just as a final note, chronic fatigue is always present. This is a condition that affects every aspect of your life and, like back problems, is hard to diagnose or prove you actually have on a constant basis. There are several factors to why I suffer from this condition, too many to repeat as most of my symptoms relate to chronic fatigue in some shape or form. Personally, it's the hardest thing I have to deal with, especially from a mental standpoint.

Speaking of mental standpoint...Let's take some time for this subject, as it is probably the hardest part of living with sarcoidosis or any other chronic health condition, for that matter. You can find a way to deal with the physical aspects, because they are there for you to feel and understand, but the mental stress is something else, especially with sarcoidosis or any other mysterious disease.

When I was first diagnosed with sarcoidosis I must admit my first reaction was relief. I had spent so many years suffering with no answer that for me to now actually have a logical explanation for the things I was feeling was a tremendous load off my mind, even if I didn't have a clue what sarcoidosis was. Hey, I wasn't crazy! To be honest, in my naive mind, I thought I would take my "replacement" medications, then aside from a little weight gain, I would be back to my normal 1986 pre-sarcoidosis lifestyle. Boy, was I in for a reality check!

The first thing I did after recovering from my hospital stay to get me adjusted to my medications was try to get back in shape and back on the basketball court. I was only 33 years old, so I still had some game left in me, at least on the YMCA level, plus this was during the Bad Boy era in Detroit (the Detroit Pistons won back-to-back NBA titles in 1989 and 1990). I had to get back to the gym and rebuild my self-esteem. Once I found out something was wrong with my pituitary gland, I told the fellows at the YMCA that I was coming back as a seven footer with the same skills I had as a six footer (the most common fact about the pituitary gland is that it controls your growth, although I've found out it does a lot more), so watch out! I spent several months slowly getting back into kinda/ sorta shape, although I knew I was easily a step slower, my quickness was not as sharp and dunking was now out of the question, as I could no longer jump over the rim…But I was still determined and naive. On my second trip back to the YMCA, reality hit me in the face.

On about the third play I made a sharp cut to the right, as my left ankle went POP! I had ripped my Achilles tendon almost in two. When I went to see my Endocrinologist a few weeks later I got a strict taste of my new reality head on, starting with him asking me, "Who told you to play full court basketball? Not me!" as he explained the reasons why I couldn't do this activity anymore. Mentally my mind was full of depression and confusion. What was I going to do now? For me basketball was more than just a game, it was a lifestyle and where I gained the majority of my personality, or so I thought. Basketball had been with me since birth. My father was a basketball coach and I even had a goal on the back of my highchair. This couldn't be happening to me! But it was.

Now I started to think like the majority of people do when they realize they have a chronic health condition that not only alters their life but also will be with them forever. I started asking myself, "Why Me?" and "What did I do to deserve this?" After spending some time depressed, but functioning and constantly asking myself, "What now?" it came to me. Having sarcoidosis and all of the other conditions was not the end of the world. I could still be happy and productive. As the saying goes "All good things come to an end". So what if my pre-sarcoidosis life had came to an end. It was now time to start a new life. I had a supportive wife and stepdaughter, along with parents who loved me unconditionally. I had a job that at this time I enjoyed (although I did get out of management due to I didn't feel it was fair to my employees for me not to be in the office on a daily basis, so I became a Business Analyst), friends, a living environment I enjoyed and I still had my health, that with proper care I could still do a lot of the things I enjoyed. Maybe it was time to enjoy some new things, but most importantly it was time to stop feeling down and move on with my life. If this was the hand God had dealt me then it was time to play the hand to win!

So at this time I put my faith as I always do in God to show me the way and started living by one of my mottos, that you will hear a lot from me, for a successful life…**Understand and honestly accept your reality then deal with it**!

This is an extremely important thing to accomplish, but don't fool yourself, it can be very difficult as well. Facing your reality in an honest manner causes you to face yourself head on and that can be an even more difficult task to accomplish. Being honest to yourself, about yourself, is easy to say, but it takes a strong person to accept it. Then once you do, you have to continue to look at yourself honestly on a daily basis because your life situations change more often than the seasons. Like reality, honesty about yourself takes courage to face and accept, but the positives you will achieve from the truth will benefit your quality of life, both physically and mentally.

The positive results you will achieve from honestly looking at your situation and also letting those people in your life understand how you feel, will bring the greatest value to your well being than anything else ever will. When you are evaluating your situation it is also extremely important to keep a positive frame of mind. The goal of this logic is for you to honestly understand what you can and cannot do, then adjust accordingly, therefore allowing you to live a happier and more productive life. Do not feel negative or less of a person when you honestly understand those things you cannot do. This is an extremely hard aspect of this process, but by doing so, you will now only focus on those things you can do instead of wasting your time and effort on things that you simply cannot do anymore, because of medical reasons. There is so much to do in life that just because one thing is ruled out doesn't stop you from doing something else.

For me not being able to play basketball, work a regular job, go somewhere at night without worrying about my diabetes insipidus and where is the nearest restroom, to play with my relatives younger kids and keep up with them, control my emotions at times; to just name a few, still causes me to sometimes feel depressed. But by accepting that those facts, among others, are now a part of my life, I can adjust accordingly and still enjoy my life, as I adjust my activities in a positive manner. I can't stress enough the importance of understanding your new reality then honestly dealing with it. To me it is the only way to go.

It will be a daily process, as I still have to look myself in the mirror every day and be honest with myself. Your life changes constantly (after all isn't that what life is, constant change?) and keeping up with those changes takes honest effort and work on your part, along with everything else you deal with. You are the only one who knows exactly what you feel. Don't go by what others think you should be feeling. Trust your own feelings and ability to determine how you feel. Trust your instincts! Facing reality can be tough, but please, for your own sake…Face your reality head on! The results will speak for themselves!

2

ME TOO!

✦

Patient Stories

Now that you've read my story, there is an important point I want to make. Although all sarcoidosis cases and results are unique, based on which organs are affected, in reality they are really all the same. I'm not alone in what I experience or in what I feel, both physically and mentally. There are many people who experience the same things as I and I'm not just talking about sarcoidosis patients, but also patients dealing with any chronic health condition. The similarities range from the physical pains, to the emotional issues of support, to the mental aspects of knowing you are chronically ill, to the many medical visits and insurance requirements; to name a few. Neither you nor I are truly alone, whether you're the patient, caregiver or friend!

To make this point I decided to get in touch with patients I knew from across the country and asked if they would donate their stories to this book. Although some didn't want their private health issues told for fear of the consequences from friends, employers, co-workers or insurance companies (which I understood/respected and is one of the reasons change/awareness needs to be improved) or some felt their lives were too boring (a point I disagreed with because any story about sarcoidosis from a patient's perspective is of value), a lot agreed to participate. First let me say "Thank You" to the patients you are about to read about and to those that weren't used in this writing for opening up their lives to me and for the world to read. It truly takes a courageous individual to be able to open up in that manner about something as private as your health and inner feelings. So if you saw yourself in some of my experiences, I'm sure you will see yourself in the following stories as well.

Margie…

I'm going to start in the San Francisco Bay area with Marguerite, who goes by the name of Margie. Margie was born in 1952 in the city of San Mateo, California. She was raised in Pacifica, California with one younger brother and an older sister in one of those houses you see on the ocean cliff, which by the way fell into the ocean in 1997 as a result of an El Nino storm. Margie had a healthy childhood, except for a bout with bronchitis when she was around five years old. She never experienced any signs of asthma or had any known allergies. A common trait you will notice in all of us is that our pre-sarcoidosis life was dramatically different than our lives today. Margie was no different.

When she was 16 years old and still in high school, Margie started professional modeling in photography, designer runway shows and on local San Francisco television. In 1970 she was crowned Miss San Francisco and Miss Photo Queen of Northern California. In 1971 while competing in the Miss California Pageant she was drawn to the excitement of the behind the scenes production work, such as the operation of the cameras and the activity in the control rooms. As she continued to model, her interest continued to be attracted to the production side of the shows as opposed to her actual modeling career, inspiring her to earn a degree in Broadcasting Arts.

Throughout the 1980s and early 1990s, Margie had a number of successful careers in television, veterinary medicine, wildlife rehabilitation, video production and Web development. Utilizing her vast experience she specialized in program development, video production and Web development for global high tech corporations as a broadcast/corporate television producer. She has produced many national live broadcast projects such as "The Lou Rawls Parade Of Stars" with Dick Clark Productions for four years and "The Easter Seals Telethon With Pat Boone" in San Francisco. In the early 1990s she started her own content development and interactive media/video production company. Margie had a great passion for life and along with her company loved animals, flying, photography and cooking. She married and has a home in the San Francisco Bay area along with a home on a working cattle ranch in Modoc County, located in Northeastern California. Life was great, at least for now.

Around 1994 Margie's good health took a downturn. She started to feel, as she terms it, "Sickly", as not only did she start to feel noticeably fatigued but in addition started to have chronic bronchitis and lung problems every winter. She saw her Primary Care Physician who basically blew the symptoms off without doing any tests and told her if she lost some weight she would be okay. This pattern continued for the next four years, every winter with the same problems and same results from her Primary Care Physician. Then in 1998 she lost sight in part of her left eye. Her Ophthalmologist thought she either had MS or a stroke. She also saw a Neurologist who did MRIs but didn't find anything out of the ordinary.

In mid-1999 she started experiencing an acute, chronic and severe cough. It quickly got to the point she couldn't complete a sentence without an explosive coughing fit. At this time she was at the height of her career and her company was doing great. However her coughing started affecting her work due to it would interrupt client meetings, shooting on location, conference calls or basically put...Everything she did. Although her customers understood and were patient with her, business is business and after a while the interruptions started costing everyone time and money. For nine months her Primary Care Physician continued prescribing antibiotics without conducting any tests to determine "what" was causing the coughing. Needless to say Margie now not only had the physical frustrations to deal with on a daily basis, but the mental and financial burdens had begun as well.

Finally in 2000, Margie and her husband demanded her Primary Care Physician, who still maintained a nonchalant attitude/approach about the cause of Margie's health problems, give her a chest X-ray to try and determine "why" she was having these problems. After all, the medications weren't helping anything so logically thinking, something aside from a temporary bug was wrong. As a result of Margie advocating for her own health and demanding that a chest X-ray be performed, she was diagnosed with pulmonary sarcoidosis, after spending six years from the time of her first symptoms back in 1994. In fact, in 2002 her Ophthalmologist admitted that she had probably had an episode with sarcoidosis in her eye back in 1998, but that was then and this is now...Four years later.

After the diagnosis and as a result of the prednisone she was now required to take on a daily basis, Margie continued to feel worse, with not much relief in sight. She was having trouble breathing due to the sarcoidosis was spreading to her lymph nodes and infiltrated into her lung tissue, which caused massive damage and inflammation. In addition the asthma attacks, chest pains, spiting up of blood from her lungs, bouts with pneumonia and weight gain from the prednisone were also contributing factors to her decline in health. For the next year and a half she was unable to work in any capacity due in large part to her hypoxia upon exertion, complications and side effects from prolonged use of prednisone, such as severe joint and muscle pain, her inability to walk any distance due to the hypoxia and weakness in her legs for support, along with edema in her feet, ankles and legs. Another factor contributing to her stamina problem was in 1990 Margie broke her right tibia and fibula requiring orthopedic surgery to fix the breaks, including inserting steel plates, screws and wires. The leg took a year to heal and actually healed offset, causing her to not be able to walk evenly on her left foot. This didn't cause any problems until she started taking prednisone. Her doctor explained prednisone will make those injured areas ache and cause small rips in her ligaments, contributing to her inability to walk long distances.

She also experiences insomnia, another side effect contributed to prednisone, along with experiencing obstructive sleep apnea, both adding to her chronic fatigue. She also believes it was a result of the prednisone that caused her to develop diabetes, hypertension and a major source for depression. Prednisone can have dramatic effects on some patients but in the same tone is needed, in most cases, to treat sarcoidosis, and in Margie's case was needed to help her breathe by allowing her to get enough air into her lungs.

However, the mental aspect and depression was caused by more than just the prednisone. As a result of her new health conditions came the financial stress of losing gainful employment and her livelihood that she worked so hard to achieve, as her customers "had" to leave her as clients in order to take care of their business (as I said earlier "business is business"), along with the inability to enjoy the things in life she loved doing such as flying airplanes, catering family functions and photography also contributed to her depression. Even her daily chores of personal care and keeping up her home suffered as she doesn't have the stamina to cook, clean, shop or just maintain a regular standard of living on her own. Let's be honest, this is a lot for one person to take!

Fortunately, she is blessed to have a supportive husband and family to help her. I can't stress enough the importance of having personal support in your life. Having a spouse who, although might not fully understand what you're experiencing from a health standpoint, does however understand that they will always be there for you, as they know you will be for them. Unfortunately we are not all as blessed, especially those who had their spouses leave them just because they couldn't handle their new health condition. That's a damn shame and one day those ex-spouses are going to need support themselves. What then? You might be healthy now but the reality of life is that it only takes a few seconds for an automobile crash to take you from a carefree healthy individual to a dependant disabled individual…Think about that for a minute! But at least for Margie and myself we are fortunate and I personally thank God everyday for that blessing!

Now her medical support has been, let's just say "Another story." Her team of medical professionals now have her on approximately 19 medications a day and at times it seems to Margie that the cure is worse than the disease. Since her diagnosis (up to 2003) she has seen 17 different doctors (not including the 10 or so that were experimental and didn't work) with a lot of hit and misses. The medical professionals included Pulmonary Specialists, Respiratory Therapists, Diabetes Specialists, Psychotherapists, Cardiology Specialists, Orthopedic Specialists, Oncologists, Infectious Disease Specialists, and Primary Care Physicians; as the list goes on! It takes a great amount of stamina (which Margie struggles to maintain) and a strong mental mind frame just to deal with the doctor trips, different results and individual doctor personalities alone. This is another example of how your doctor and their staff treat their patients makes such a difference in the patient's outlook. This is why the little things really do make a difference!

With sarcoidosis in her lungs, eyes and now the doctors think in her bronchial tubes and trachea, both the physical demands and mental stress can at times be overwhelming. But by keeping a positive attitude, advocating for herself, having a supportive husband and doing whatever she can to understand everything she can about her disease, Margie continues to survive and strive for the quality of life she deserves.

On the bright side, her doctors feel the sarcoidosis has for now stopped infiltrating into her lungs. They feel it's her bronchial tubes and trachea that's exacerbating the asthma she has developed as a result of sarcoidosis. So they have now started the first phases of reducing her intake of prednisone and hopefully will reduce the negative side effects of the drug…A positive roller coaster for Margie to ride into the future. In fact, in the first two months she has lost 35 pounds and as a result Margie is now off oxygen. As Margie put it, "I now have this renewed fire in my belly to get healthy!"

During our discussions I asked Margie a couple of questions. First I asked, "What is your biggest fear and hope in life?" She replied, "My biggest fear is that I will slowly get worse and no matter what I do, the disease will make me an invalid who has to depend on others for my care. I fear that I will slowly die or have complications that cause me to die an early death." This is a normal response that I hear a lot of and one we all must deal with in our own way.

She went on to say, "My greatest hope is that with the knowledge and involvement in my healing with both western and alternative medicine, I will get better and be able to resume the life I so anxiously want to do again. My passion for life and all that I have been involved in has taught me that there are many opportunities around and if you can be open to them, you can live some wonderful life experiences. I wish more than anything I could enjoy these life experiences, no matter where in the world it might take me and my husband."

Next I asked, "What message would like to leave from your story?" Margie replied, "If there is one sore point I would like to leave with people it's that, in my opinion, the medical profession is not as proactive as you would like or expect. I find with this managed care stuff, they don't have or do not want to spend the extra time figuring out what is really wrong with you. If you don't fit into the typical categories, many doctors blow off your symptoms and tell you that you are either imagining it or inventing it or it is because I'm fat. And what you really need is someone to help you get back to normal health. Western medicine is a science of surgeries and chemicals. They give a pill or a procedure for everything. They don't look at the whole person. I have found that you have to be your own advocate and get knowledgeable about your disease and how to treat it. I would say the Traditional Chinese Medicine and metaphysical work in Buddhist Mindfulness Meditations have helped me as much, if not more, than the western drugs. I also believe in visualization to see myself healthy and my lungs working well and "will" my body to be better. I say all this, but I am remiss in practicing all these things the way I should. I think my depression has contributed to getting so tired of trying to heal myself, so that I don't keep up on it like I should."

When I asked in closing what pointers she felt were important for others to follow, based on her experience as a patient, she responded, "Advocate for yourself, keep all your test results, know your medications and their side effects, try to keep a list of everything that goes on with your health and how you feel then take those notes to your doctor visits, learn breathing techniques, ask for help and most importantly remember who you are because being sick with sarcoidosis will eventually make you feel as if this is all you do in life and your life is far too valuable for that kind of attitude!" Well said!

Chris...

Chris was born in 1962 and raised in Trenton, Michigan. Trenton is a suburb of Detroit located in an area known to the locals as "downriver". It's primarily a middle class, blue collar suburb and like the majority of metro Detroit in that era depended largely on the automotive industry for its economic success. Chris was the sixth of seven children and grew up in a stable household. He was fortunate to be raised by two loving parents. Being brought up in an environment of unconditional love instilled fortitude and strength of character in Chris. He was a shy kid who stayed out of trouble and only had a few close friends, although if you can honestly say you have a few close friends then you are doing just fine. He enjoyed both baseball and hockey, but because of his shyness never tried out for any of the organized leagues. Like most Detroiters he remains a loyal Detroit sports fan to this day, something I personally can appreciate, although at the time of this writing (Winter 2004) that takes guts to say in regard to our beloved Lions (NFL). But if you've ever been a Detroit sports fan then you know what we mean!

Chris went on to earn his degree at Western Michigan University in Kalamazoo, Michigan. He moved to Dallas, Texas in 1984 searching for employment, as the job market in metro Detroit at the time was tight. He worked for a few different companies before settling into long-term employment. In 1987 his current employer hired him and he has been with the company ever since. He briefly married a Texas woman in 1986 but they both quickly realized their marriage was not going to work, for reasons other than health related issues, as Chris was still in excellent health at the time. In 1993 Chris was transferred to San Diego, California and met his current wife in 1994. This time around everything is working out just fine.

From a health perspective Chris had always been in exceptional health. Except for the normal cold or growing aches and pains, he never experienced any unusual health problems as a child, teenager or adult. He was one of those individuals who never worried about his health, although he did seem to have more kidney stones that the average person. However, even though they were painful, they never slowed him down and he enjoyed life to the fullest without a health care worry in the world. He had worked his way up the corporate ladder, doing something he enjoyed, with a company he had been with for some time and had a wife who as he put it, "Is an incredible human being"…So in other words his life couldn't have been better. But then came the Christmas holiday season of 1999!

Just before the Christmas holiday his ankles swelled and he started experiencing pains in his joints throughout his body. In addition, he started to experience severe fatigue, a persistent cough and was having a hard time breathing. He went to see his regular doctor at the time who, without running any tests, concluded his salt intake was too high, which was causing his sudden problems. This seemed strange to Chris since his diet hadn't changed in years nor had his salt intake increased. In fact, nothing in his lifestyle had changed for some time. This not only frustrated Chris but frustrated his wife as well.

Shortly after the beginning of the year 2000, as the symptoms continued to worsen, his wife insisted that he see her doctor, since even after a second visit with the same complaints, his doctor didn't seem to want to pursue "what" was really causing her husband's problems. Like I've written many times…It's your health at stake so if you aren't getting the support you think you deserve then find another doctor who is willing to at least try and help you. There are too many good caring doctors available to waste your time and worsen your health with a doctor you are uncomfortable with. We can't expect a medical professional of any type to know every time what is wrong with us, but we can expect them to at least try to understand and if they don't know then ask for help. How many times have we seen examples of this? Anyway…She made an appointment for Chris with her doctor and after explaining Chris's symptoms, his wife asked or shall I say demanded, the doctor perform a chest X-ray. She had heard that swollen ankles could be indicative of a heart problem and that concerned not only her but Chris as well, so the doctor agreed. It turned out to be a great move not to waste any time on the previous doctor, as that's a mistake a lot of us (myself included) have made during our pre-diagnosis period. As a result of this chest X-ray the ball started rolling to determine "what" was causing Chris's problems.

What appeared on the chest X-ray seemed to be swollen lymph nodes so the doctor ordered a CAT scan, which confirmed the lymph nodes were considerably enlarged. It was a result of this report that the diagnosis of sarcoidosis was first mentioned as a possible cause for Chris's health problems. In addition there was some visible lung scarring and skin lesions, so the doctor referred Chris to a lung specialist for further tests and to confirm his suspicions of sarcoidosis as the cause. A positive example of a doctor immediately asking for help, which again as patients is all we ask!

With the symptoms Chris had been experiencing everyone suspected sarcoidosis, but the doctor stated that lymphoma was also a possibility, so at this point the testing moved rapidly. First, a bronchoschopy was performed but proved inconclusive. So at this time he was sent to a surgeon to have a mediastinoscopy performed to biopsy Chris's lymph nodes. It was at this point the diagnosis of sarcoidosis was confirmed.

As mentioned earlier, Chris seemed to have a more than usual number of kidney stones but after the diagnosis he really started producing a lot of kidney stones very rapidly. He now passed a minimum of several each year and they were excruciating each and every time…Something you never get used to! In hindsight, as a result of the sarcoidosis now determined as the cause for his many kidney stones, along with his history of suffering from stones for quite a few years, the doctors suspect Chris may have had sarcoidosis for several years prior to the official diagnosis. In part due to his multiple relocations over the previous years, it was hard for his doctors to have a continuous history on his medical background, so the connection was never considered until the ankle swelling incident and chest X-ray. Regardless of how many times you move around or change doctors and no matter how difficult, costly or frustrating it is to obtain your medical records, I can't stress the importance of being able to give your medical professionals your complete and honest medical history and present symptoms. This is the only way they are going to be able to determine exactly what is wrong with you in a timely manner, and as we've seen many times, a timely manner can have a dramatic effect on your life and those around you!

Since Chris's diagnosis, he has had to have a few stays in the hospital due to blockages and kidney infection. On occasion his medical professionals have had to use a scope to smash and remove the kidney stones in the urethra. Sarcoidosis can cause high concentrations of calcium in the urine and/or blood. In Chris's case, he has high amounts of calcium in his urine, but not in his blood. The year 2003 was pretty good, as Chris only passed five or six kidney stones, for him a small number, for anyone else, too many. During the first year after his diagnosis, he also developed hemorrhoids and had excruciating sinus infections, both probably due to and certainly at least exacerbated by swelling caused by the sarcoidosis. To help with the sinus problem, Chris had surgery in 2001 to open up his sinus. The procedure consisted of basically cutting out much of the swollen tissue. However, to this day he experiences nose bleeds on a regular basis. As with most of us, he just deals with the hemorrhoids.

Like us all, Chris's life has changed considerably after he was diagnosed with sarcoidosis in 2000. He currently sees several specialists on a regular basis, such as a Pulmonologist, Urologist, Gastroenterologist, Dermatologist, and Rheumatologist. Other specialists are seen as needed, and then of course there is his family doctor. His Rheumatologist has turned out to be the specialist who was both the most well-versed in treating sarcoidosis, and the most instrumental in improving Chris's quality of life, so he functions as Chris's Primary Physician. In today's medical environment you sometimes need a palm pilot to keep track of them all.

However his biggest battle, both physically and mentally, is with the chronic fatigue that is always present. As Chris puts it, "It is so debilitating. Plus there are times when I literally can't get out of bed for days, occasionally sleeping as many as 24-30 hours straight through. But what can you do?" I wish I knew the answer to that question! As I've mentioned many times chronic fatigue is something that will not only wear on you physically but primarily mentally, especially when your pre-sarcoidosis life was spent active and with the liberty to do the things you enjoyed without giving energy or fatigue a second thought.

The sarcoidosis that affects his lungs seems to be improving over the past year, as his breathing has become better. But now, in addition to the fatigue and kidney stones, arthritis has become a serious fight for Chris, something that had never been an issue prior to his diagnosis of sarcoidosis. The sarcoidosis has attacked his joints with a vengeance. Although traditional arthritis treatments such as Enbrel (an at home injectable medication) help somewhat, the only thing that really improves it dramatically is large doses of steroids. But, after having had several runs of steroids in the past few years, he has now developed osteoporosis, so now steroids can only be taken sparingly. In addition, Chris developed skin lesions that resemble symptoms of erythema, an abnormal redness of the skin due to capillary congestion and lichen planus, which are autoimmune diseases characterized by papular eruptions most commonly on the extremities. Add the fact that having one autoimmune disease can make additional autoimmune diseases, or for that matter additional secondary chronic health conditions more likely, the mental stress of dealing with that thought can be a heavy load for anyone.

Fortunately, Chris has the support of his wife and friends, something that makes an extremely positive difference in a patient's life. His wife, who also has a chronic illness of her own, has not only been understanding and supportive, but as we saw earlier, involved with the process Chris has been going through during his sarcoidosis experience. Although his family and friends can't truly understand exactly what Chris deals with on an ever-present daily basis or for that matter might not even understand what sarcoidosis really is or the actual effect it has on his life, they are supportive and that's really all we as patients can ask of those around us. So in that aspect Chris is a lucky man!

When he was first diagnosed with sarcoidosis his employer supported him 100%. But as time goes on and living with sarcoidosis becomes an every day struggle, it hasn't been so easy. He recently took a leave of absence (short term disability) due to a bout with the most severe fatigue he has experienced to date, along with dealing with stomach issues as well. It got to the point he literally couldn't hold food down for several weeks straight. As a result Chris was hospitalized for several days before being sent home and put on intravenous feeding for a few weeks.

His boss moved on approximately two years ago and the new boss's tolerance for illness is much lower than that of his previous boss. His job reviews have deteriorated and his boss has made comments to the effect of, "You were not missed while you were out on leave." This has been devastating for Chris, to say the least, especially for a career employee of 16 years who had always excelled in all previous years. This is a heavy mental and emotional burden for anyone to bear, as he tries harder to find out how this person wants him to perform his job duties.

Unfortunately, this is a problem most sarcoidosis patients or for that matter, anyone with a chronic health condition has to endure. I understand business is business, but a loyal employee should not be made to suffer just because they have a chronic health condition. There are ways to tap into that employee's vast experience and loyalty and continue to get positive results and production from the employee. Plus, from a business aspect it's cheaper and more productive to keep experienced employees than it is to hire and train new ones. Of course, when you hire a new employee you usually pay them less and when an employee uses benefits it takes a toll on the bottom line as well.

Most employees spend more time on the job than they do waking hours at home; therefore how they are treated makes a major difference in their lives. To make matters worse, it's always amazing to me how a healthy person reacts to how a person with a chronic health condition should perform on the job, as if they are lazy or for some reason lost all of the experience and skills they once had. If employers, or more specifically people who have a "little" power over some-one's career would treat that employee as they would like to be treated, then we wouldn't have a need for laws such as the Americans with Disability Act (ADA)…But unfortunately we do. This is just a fact of life that needs to be addressed over and over again, and not in just Chris's case, but for many chroni-cally ill patients who can still perform their jobs in the same productive manner, if given a fair chance.

For Chris and many others, their careers are important to them. Not only does it help make them still feel productive, the health insurance alone makes keeping their jobs, regardless of how they feel, a necessity. His battles with sarcoidosis should not be topped with a battle to keep his job in which he is still productive. But as my saying goes, "Reality is reality and we must do what we have to do!" But Chris will be fine because he has a positive attitude, loving wife, supportive friends and a team of specialists who are willing to now look at "what" causes his symptoms. So like all of us with sarcoidosis, Chris will continue to, "Live one day at a time and keep his head to the sky!" When it comes down to it…What else can we really do?

Carol…

Let's now visit South Carolina and Carol. When I was going through the process of writing/publishing "*ME & SARCOIDOSIS—A LIFETIME PARTNER-*

SHIP", I wanted to do everything myself. It was a matter of principle for me because I didn't want any outside influence to alter my story just to sell more books. It was my objective to bring awareness to sarcoidosis by way of my experiences and story. Well, needless to say, I made a lot of rookie mistakes. A primary mistake was not getting a professional proofreader, but instead trusting someone else, while I handled other aspects of getting the book published, who was not qualified to handle a project the size of my book. As a result the initial book released contained numerous editing problems that were not discovered until several hundred copies into production, thus the reason for the wording "Revised Edition" on the cover of the book you see today. Now, once I was made aware of the problems, I immediately took responsibility for the problems and revised the book. This is when I met Carol.

I met Carol by way of SarcoidBuddies in 2002, an online chat support group discussed in detail later in this book, as I was explaining and apologizing to any members who might have purchased the mistake-ridden version of my first book. Although the story and message was not damaged, the ease of reading the book could cause readers to become frustrated, although I've had many readers who have told me they never even noticed the mistakes because they were so into my story. Carol immediately spoke up and volunteered her proofreading services to me since she had previously been a technical proofreader. I took her up on her offer and will never forget the professional assistance, encouragement and personal advice she provided me on not only my first book, but this project as well. So for that I want to publicly say, "Thank you Carol!"

Carol was born in 1949 and raised in Newark, New Jersey until she was 20 years old. While growing up she spent many weekends around the coal mines and coal hills in the Dunmore (Scranton), Pennsylvania area visiting her grandparents. In addition, for most of her early years the family home was heated by burning coal during the cold New Jersey winters. To add to the environmental situation during this time, that area of New Jersey was known for its heavy industrial contaminants, many to which Carol might have been exposed.

When she was around nine years old she developed a chronic cough. Now back in those days and environment you never went to see a doctor for a cough! Finally after nine months and the chronic cough still present, her mother took her to see the "neighborhood" doctor. He claimed that since she was beginning to go through the puberty years it was probably just a "nervous tic". After that time she often had periods of swollen glands and unexplainable times of developing pneumonia. Looking back and in hindsight this could have very easily been when

Carol first developed sarcoidosis. Unfortunately that's something we will never know! She eventually ended up in South Carolina with her husband.

Her diagnosis for sarcoidosis was probably unusual, even for sarcoidosis patients. In July 1999 Carol went through surgery for stage I breast cancer. She had a small malignant lump in her left breast and at the time her doctor told her that she was one of the best candidates for survival he had ever met due to the fact she had great counts on everything tested. After her surgery, radiation and chemotherapy treatments were still going to be needed. As soon as she started her radiation treatments, which focused strongly on the upper lobe of the left lung, Carol began to feel horrible and drained, even more than normal for individuals going through the same treatment.

After her second chemotherapy session she experienced a very bad night and had to be taken to the emergency room at the medical center where she was being treated. At that time a chest X-ray was taken and she was re-hydrated. The next day her Oncologist called and told her that her chest X-ray came back "fuzzy". She was immediately scheduled for a CAT scan, for which she agreed, not realizing how serious this could be. Several days later her Oncologist informed her that she had multiple lesions in her lungs, and in her case, it could very well be stage IV breast cancer that had spread to her lungs! Carol and her husband went home devastated with this news. She proceeded to make plans for her funeral. Carol was only 50 years old at the time.

Upon the recommendation of her Oncologist, she continued with her chemotherapy to treat her breast cancer along with continuing to get CAT scans. The CAT scans continued to show the lesions in her lungs would abate and then show up again. Carol truly felt that it was breast cancer cells that had metastasized.

Eventually, the spots in her lungs went away and she felt she was free and clear of the breast cancer! She finally felt relief…The lesions were gone! But, after her eighth chemotherapy treatment, her Oncologist suggested that they perform yet another lung and liver scan; just to as they put it, "Make sure that everything was okay." Well, it wasn't! All of the lesions were back in the lungs. Again, the funeral plans were on high alert!

Carol was finally referred to a Pulmonologist. He performed spirometry tests, more CAT scans (including High RES), and a bronchoschopy, which Carol later commented, "That was not a very comfortable test at all!" The results were a toss-up between the doctors. They couldn't decide if she was having an allergic reaction to the methotrexate part of her chemotherapy treatments or if there was a possibility it might be sarcoidosis. Either way Carol wanted to find out what was wrong now, not later. And by the way, "What the heck is sarcoidosis?"

Confusion and frustration now was setting in even more, although she was extremely relieved it wasn't stage IV breast cancer to her lungs. But if it wasn't cancer then what was it? This was a question Carol asked over and over as another year came and went. Of course, now in hindsight, we know it was sarcoidosis.

It wasn't until then that Carol's blood tests started showing her liver counts to be a lot higher than the acceptable range. At this time she had surgery to remove her gall bladder. Being proactive, Carol suggested that while they were in there for the surgery why not do a liver biopsy? The doctors agreed and performed the liver biopsy and the results were not what Carol wanted to hear!

Turns out she had stage III-IV cirrhosis of the liver, fatty liver, and several other liver problems, all due to the sarcoidosis. Based on how her liver looked from the outside due to the sarcoidosis, the surgeon informed her, "In my opinion, you will probably need a liver transplant within two years." However when she went to the liver specialist he told her, "We can't put you on the liver transplant list until May 2005 due to the fact we must wait five years after your chemotherapy before we could perform a transplant."

I believe this is a common misconception in regard to how sarcoidosis looks to some in the medical profession. When I was in the hospital in 1991 to adjust me to my new medications as I had just been diagnosed with sarcoidosis, they did a chest X-ray on my lungs. The technician actually ran to my Pulmonologist to let him know he had a terminally ill patient on his hands and he had verified it with another doctor. They concluded that based on how my lungs looked I wasn't going to make it much longer if something wasn't done immediately. Fortunately by then my doctors knew it was sarcoidosis and told the technician it was okay, they had it under control...Thank God! But for Carol this was not good news at all and is something she must live with for now! If only she had been diagnosed with sarcoidosis earlier, but again that seems to be a common statement made after the fact in regard to sarcoidosis...Case after case. This is my main argument as to why priority needs to be given to develop standard and routine tests that are run on a regular basis to detect sarcoidosis in its early stages instead of waiting on a biopsy!

Now, as with us all, I believe it's the mental aspect of having sarcoidosis that is the most difficult and Carol was no different. Her family and friends still can't manage to spell sarcoidosis, except for her, as she describes him, "Hang-in-there husband!" If there is one statement worth repeating over and over again from a patient's perspective it's, "What a difference positive support from our spouse makes in our life!" Sarcoidosis still seems so alien to people, including some in the medical profession, as some of Carol's doctors seemed uncomfortable with the terminology of the disease (this is something I can testify to as well).

She does, however, credit her dentist as someone who made a point to understand how sarcoidosis could affect what he was doing. When Carol went for a normal checkup and told her dentist about her newfound health condition, he readily admitted he didn't know what sarcoidosis was. When she returned for her follow-up for the needed dental work, the dentist informed the technician all about sarcoidosis and exactly what Carol was dealing with, including making it a point to instruct the technician to be very gentle. It was obvious the dentist had done his homework! What's funny is that I experienced a similar situation with a dental professional.

In my case I was getting an initial examination by a gum specialist to determine what was needed due to my increasing gum problems. After the examination the Periodontist left the room for quite a long time. I thought he was probably just taking care of another patient or reviewing X-rays and such since waiting is a norm for any area of the medical profession. But when he returned he apologized for taking so long and explained that he was reading his research books to make sure he had an understanding of how sarcoidosis could affect my teeth and gums, although he also added, "There really wasn't much information to be found." But like Carol, I really appreciated and respected the fact he admitted he wasn't sure how sarcoidosis affected what he was going to do and took the time to research to make sure he did understand "before" he made any determinations or actions regarding my dental issues. If only everyone would be as honest and professional!

Carol is normally an upbeat and very positive person, but during the times of her tests and uncertainties she found herself crying much of the time and laying in bed with the covers pulled over her head trying to hide from all the exhaustion she was constantly feeling. Dealing with cancer, then being told it has likely spread to your lungs, then to your liver, the fatigue, the non-comprehending looks from your family and peers after the sarcoidosis diagnosis (after all, at least it's NOT cancer again, was their refrain!), well, it all becomes quite overwhelming for a person to handle.

The mental aspect of any type of chronic disease, both during and after the diagnosis periods, can be tremendous. It's extremely important that you find your own way of dealing with it head on or it can destroy you. Another reason I stress to understand your reality, honestly accept it then deal with it in the best way that fits your personality and lifestyle…PLEASE!

In 2003 Carol had to go in for another mammogram, which showed a "string of suspicious cells at the site of the original tumor" and had a follow-up breast biopsy performed. The June 2003 biopsy results were benign. However, that biopsy site resulted in an enlarged cyst in her left breast, which was drained in December 2003. After the procedure was performed, she has been given different opinions as to what to expect. Her sarcoidosis specialist told her, "Sarcoidosis granulomas just 'love' scar tissue." He believed her "re-current" breast cancer scare was likely sarcoidosis granulomas from the scar tissue. He stressed that it didn't matter if it was sarcoidosis, all breast lumps need to have a biopsy performed because of the possibility of it actually being a malignancy, especially in the case of Carol and her past history with breast cancer, radiation and chemotherapy treatments. On the other hand, her Radiologist thinks it's cancer...Period. So is it sarcoidosis spreading or is it cancer spreading? Carol ended up having two breast biopsies performed in just six months. As of this writing Carol has been dealing with these same issues, questions and procedures for five years and as she puts it, "I'm so worn out!" I believe anyone would feel that way!

After being diagnosed with liver disease in 2002, upon the advice of her surgeon, Carol decided it was time to find out about Social Security disability. A word of advice from everyone I know who has filed for Social Security...If you feel that you have any case at all, apply immediately! In her case (as in many, many, many, many others) it took Social Security nine months to officially turn her down, even though per the Social Security's criteria it stated if you have a bilirubin count of 2.5 or above for three months in a row, you qualify for disability benefits. Now keep in mind Carol exceeded this requirement, as it had now been nine months, however she was still rejected. In the eyes of Social Security and other insurance policies as well, sarcoidosis primarily only causes you shortness of breath, minor joint pains and slight fatigue. I've seen this explanation on more than one occasion even though each case is different and it's the secondary conditions caused by sarcoidosis that are the problem. Just another reason for the need for a broader legal definition of sarcoidosis!

So, as I personally would recommend doing "before" ever even filing your claim, Carol hired an attorney. But there was another common problem she faced...Her husband's COBRA coverage was to end soon and to qualify for Medicare (except in extreme cases) you have to be officially approved for Social Security for 24 months, a policy that makes absolutely no sense to me. To my simple mind, if you qualify for disability, don't you need health insurance at that time, not 24 months later? So technically, regardless of her Social Security decision, Carol was going to be without health insurance for the next six months. A financial disaster for anyone with a chronic health condition!

Another option she has was that she could apply to the South Carolina State Health Insurance Pool, to the tune of $838 a month for her alone! There is a $500 deductible along with a lot of other clauses that all far exceed what you can afford on the monthly income you get from Social Security…Even if you get the maximum. It amazes me to hear healthy people say how those on Social Security are lazy or just wanting to get one over on the system. Do they realize how much you actually get compared to what you could make on even a low paying non-skilled job? You don't get rich on Social Security and for most people I know your quality of living from a financial standpoint goes down, quite a bit, not to mention you have been paying into the system your entire working life. But your health is the most important thing to your survival so you do what you have to do!

One thing Carol stressed to me based on her experiences was this, "Having breast cancer is very presentable to the general population. Everyone has heard of this disease and I have been swimming in that breast cancer pool for four years now—and it can be overwhelming. However, very few people have heard of sarcoidosis and that is probably the disease that is most devastating to me right now of the two. I am so truly exhausted with fighting the Social Security system in dealing with the reasons why I should be termed "disabled" at the appropriate time. The people who make these decisions about us are completely healthy people who have not dealt with debilitating issues that wear us out on a regular basis, making such life-bearing decisions that make me worry on a day-to-day basis, such as what operation I should elect to have or what prescription should be filled. Something needs to change!" Amen to that, as I'm sure there are many of us that can relate!

In the meantime she maintains a positive attitude about the fact she has a very unusual unpronounceable disease and she does everything she can to keep her head from under the covers so that she can face life head on. Aside from using the Internet to chat with other sarcoidosis patients, one of her main joys is doing volunteer work at her Cancer Center's gift shop. She feels she helps new patients who come in as they share stories and she can show them living proof that you can still be alive four plus years after you have dealt with death defying health issues and ongoing drama. This is a lesson we can all learn from!

Dan...

Dan was born in 1970 and raised in the rural upstate New York town of Chester. Chester is the type of town where everyone knows your name and during Dan's childhood, hardly anyone ever moved in or out, a very stable environment. During his childhood he worked on his neighbor's produce farm, harvesting lettuce and onions. His childhood was rather normal and aside from a large number of sinus infections on a yearly basis, he was in good health. In fact, as he put it, "I never even had a broken bone."

Dan joined the Air Force right out of high school. He was trained on how to repair electronic systems on F-15 fighter jets. After completing his term of duty, he went on to work for a major airline in Dallas, Texas and, as of this writing, is still employed with the company.

For pleasure Dan got his own private pilot's license to fly helicopters. In his pre-sarcoidosis days he was very active, enjoying such activities as water and snow skiing, indoor rock climbing, yard work and major remodeling projects around the house (a talent I sure could use around my home, as my wife takes care of our remodeling projects!). Dan was never afraid to knock down a wall or tear out the kitchen. "In fact, the final product was usually better than I had originally planned", Dan told me proudly. But as the stories have all gone, that all changed as his good health took a turn for the worse.

It was the night of January 30, 2000, the same night of the Super Bowl in which the St. Louis Rams beat the Tennessee Titans, and Dan's heater broke. He awoke the next morning freezing, as he seriously/jokingly puts it to this Detroit resident, "Yes, it does get cold in Dallas." Once he got the heater fixed he noticed he had developed a cough, but just thought it was a normal cold, as his doctor just prescribed an antibiotic and he continued to go about his normal business. After about a month and continuing to cough, he went back to the doctor. This time around he was diagnosed with pneumonia and given another round of antibiotics and cough drops. Three weeks later the only change was now Dan was coughing to the point of losing his breath, so back to his doctor for the third time.

This time a chest X-ray was performed, which came back showing something on Dan's lungs. The doctor told Dan that he might have cancer and then performed some blood tests to send to the lab. Dan went home to wait for the results. Needless to say, this was a very stressful period of what seemed like everlasting time from a mental perspective for Dan, as it would be for anyone. Well, the results came back negative for cancer, good news except...Now the doctor told Dan he might have AIDS. From the possibility of cancer to AIDS…What a mental roller coaster? After a couple of sleepless nights, the results again came back negative, good news again but at the same time it raised the question of "what" was that something on Dan's lungs causing him to continue to cough to the point of causing shortness of breath and for such an extended period of time?

So Dan was referred to a Pulmonologist who performed a bronchoschopy and took a biopsy from his lung. As a result of those tests and after four months of non-stop coughing, medications, X-rays, blood tests, mental stress and multiple doctor visits, Dan was diagnosed with sarcoidosis. Like most of us Dan's first response was, "I've got what?" His Pulmonologist told him that most people who had sarcoidosis ended up getting better within about two years and he really shouldn't worry about it. I wish I knew where these medical professionals get that statistic or logic and I wish even more they would keep it to themselves. This is one of the problems we face when patients try to get help, such as disability bene-fits, because the denial comes back as if sarcoidosis is no big deal and will just go. Well, it is a big deal and it just doesn't affect the lungs for a couple of years then just go away. I guarantee you the percentage of patients that it "just goes away" doesn't come remotely close to the comparison to the patients who suffer with the disease for life, and definitely not just from a lung standpoint. Show me that statistic! It's time to get away from that misleading logic because it only hurts sar-coidosis patients that need help. Okay, back to Dan.

Although he kept hoping the Pulmonologist was right, after all over the next couple of years he only experienced the normal sinus infections, colds and very small bouts with skin rashes, nothing to get worked up about. But the reality was, the Pulmonologist was wrong. In the fall of 2002 a small lump appeared on Dan's forehead, similar to a normal "zit". Only it lasted for a few months and if you squeezed it nothing came out…Not a normal "zit"! Dan's girlfriend (now his wife) referred him to a plastic surgeon who removed the lump with no problem. However, when it came back from the lab (it's normal procedure when a lump is removed to send it for testing), it came back as sarcoidosis. As expected, everyone was shocked! "Wasn't the sarcoidosis just in my lungs and no big deal?" Dan asked.

Dan went back to the Pulmonologist who performed lung function tests, blood work and a chest X-ray, but nothing seemed out of the ordinary, so they decided to monitor the situation closely for the next few months.

The year 2003 started out good for Dan. His personal life was on the path he had always hoped to be on when he turned 33 and he was in love with the woman who he now planned to marry. Plus, he hadn't heard any bad news from the monitoring of his sarcoidosis, so maybe life would be great again after all. Unfortunately, this turning point in Dan's life turned the wrong way.

It started with another sinus infection and another dose of antibiotics. Then he started having severe diarrhea that lasted for about 11 days. He went to the doctor on day four, then back again on day eight. Finally on day 10 he was referred to a specialist. By this time his body was shutting down and the medications were having no effect, so he was admitted to the hospital, even though everyone around him kept telling him, "You don't look sick." After a few more days of antibiotics, along with diarrhea, the doctors diagnosed him with pseudo membranous colitis, also known as antibiotic induced colitis, and can appear after being on antibiotics for a long period of time. Antibiotics were the usual medication prescribed Dan for his sinus infections and such.

Over the next few days, Dan began to feel better, except for a pain in his right lower back near his hip. In about a week the diarrhea reappeared so the doctors decided to perform a colonoscopy to look for colon disease. Nothing was found during the colonoscopy, so they performed more X-rays to look for "what" was causing the pain. As a result they found Dan's problem to be arthritis in his hip joint. Over the next three months Dan dealt with the pain with over the counter pain pills, then the pain progressively worsened in a very short time. He started taking a low dose prescription pain pill, and within a week, had to move up to a narcotic pain prescription.

Dan had a good relationship with his family doctor, a major plus when dealing with chronic health conditions, as they decided to again X-ray both the hip and pelvic areas to look for any advancements of the arthritis. The next day a call came with the X-ray results and more disturbing news. The arthritis was the same, but there was a tumor on his L-4 vertebrae. "A tumor on my spine", Dan thought with worry. "I had watched both of my grandmothers die from cancer. All I could think was that it was my turn", he confessed. So an MRI of Dan's spine was ordered.

As a result of the MRI, it was found that the bone marrow of Dan's vertebrae and hips were full of something. The term leukemia was mentioned, and by this time as Dan put it, "I was ready to get off of this roller coaster!" Luckily his girlfriend remembered Dan's skin and lung sarcoidosis, and asked if this could be related. The Radiologist said that bone sarcoidosis is rare, but it could explain this situation. Only a bone marrow biopsy would tell us what it was. It's a good thing Dan's girlfriend remembered the sarcoidosis because otherwise that would never have been thought of, at least for quite a while and who knows after what other symptoms. Another example of advocating for your own health, or in this case, making sure your primary caregiver is aware of all your health situations.

Dan's father had donated bone marrow to his uncle a few years earlier, and everything was a success. So he figured that since this was just to take a sample, it shouldn't be a big deal. Well, when you pull up to a Cancer Institute, reality starts to set in. I experienced the same feeling when I took a loved one for an appointment for the first time. It hadn't really hit me how serious she was until we entered the building with the sign "Cancer Treatment Center" by the door. Don't fool yourself…No matter what is wrong with you, if you're at a Cancer Institute, it's a big deal!

When the time came for the procedure to begin, Dan was given a medicine lollypop, or commonly known as a "morphine lollypop". During the procedure Dan was conscious, as they bore a hole in his hipbone, and took a sample of the bone and the marrow. With the "morphine lollypop" doing its thing, all Dan felt was pressure. He was cracking jokes throughout the procedure. The doctor and nurses thought it was the medicine, but anyone who knows Dan knows that's how he deals with tough times. Laughter and being able to laugh at yourself or situation is great therapy. As they say, "It takes more muscles to frown than it does to smile." There is a reason we were created that way…Think about it.

A couple of days later the test results came back negative for cancer and positive for sarcoidosis. Dan thought to himself, "Okay, here I am diagnosed with vertebral sarcoidosis. A 33 year old male, who according to everything I've been told about sarcoidosis, doesn't fit any of the stereotypes and everyone I come in contact with tells me "I don't look sick". Who came up with these stereotypes in the first place and I sure wish I felt like I looked!"

Upon doing his research, with limited information available, Dan found that sarcoidosis of the bone occurs in about 5% of people with the disease, usually in the hands. But sarcoidosis of the vertebrae is very rare. Dan found a sarcoidosis specialist in Dallas, but since vertebral sarcoidosis is so rare, he hadn't dealt with it before. This was something Dan expected, and still was comfortable with the specialist, as to Dan he seemed very competent. At least he was honest, which again is all we as patients really ask from our medical professionals.

Dan started a course of high dose corticosteroids or more specifically, prednisone, and started to feel less pain. The doctors think that he will probably be on the high doses for a while, and possibly be on a lower maintenance dose for at least a year. Due to the advanced involvement with his bone marrow, high doses of prednisone shouldn't be used for a long period of time. High doses of prednisone for a long period of time may cause bone loss or osteoporosis. When the bones are involved, the sarcoidosis can cause bone loss as well. A Catch 22 if there ever was one.

In August 2003 Dan started methotrexate and lowered his intake of prednisone. Methotrexate is an immuno-suppressive therapy. They used to call it chemotherapy, but Dan's guess is they didn't want to scare everyone these days so they changed the name. In sarcoidosis patients the doses are lower than in cancer patients, and usually the side effects are less severe.

Well, in a couple of months after the start of methotrexate, whereas they started Dan at a low dose then tapered up to try to avoid any major side effects, there weren't any noticeable side effects as he reached 15MG per week, where the doctor is hoping to maintain him. As the methotrexate was increased, he decreased the prednisone, which was now at 60MG per day. To prevent shocking the adrenal system you have to decrease prednisone intake slowly, so they decreased Dan's by 10MG per day, then maintain that level for a week. If everything seemed to be going well, then the prednisone level would decrease again.

Dan made it down to 20MG per day before the lower back and hip pain started to return. He spoke with his specialist, and he recommended increasing the prednisone dose back to 30MG. By the next week, the pain was incredible once again. As a result Dan was back on the narcotics.

As the pain persisted, the prednisone had to continue to be increased until Dan was back up to the 60MG original dosage, as the pain just won't seem to go away. In addition, the pain medication has been increased as well, although there are still times when that doesn't seem to help much either. Everyone keeps hoping the methotrexate will start suppressing the sarcoidosis soon. The steroid level can't be kept this high for much longer without running the risk of other problems. So for now Dan just keeps cracking jokes and praying.

Throughout this journey Dan has received unconditional support from his spouse, both as his girlfriend and as his wife. In addition his friends, co-workers and employer have shown him nothing but positive support, although they still think "he doesn't look sick" and have a hard time understanding what exactly Dan goes through with this "sarcoidosis thing". Join the club—because even us with the disease have a hard time understanding at times and we live with it. Then finding information regarding our disease can be even more frustrating for us and those we love who want to understand what we are dealing with. Thus, Dan had an idea.

He formed a non-profit organization, which he named **Sarcoid Life**, to try to help educate people about sarcoidosis. Dan felt that information about sarcoidosis was so spread out and fragmented among different sources making reliable or useful information hard to find. He wanted to create one organization that would combine this information and keep it as current as possible for other sarcoidosis patients, their families, friends, co-workers and most of all, physicians. Since in reality, physicians are taught very little about sarcoidosis, he could help provide a resource tool that could assist in the treatment methods of sarcoidosis patients. By making the information readily available via the Internet and in one location, it would help the physicians stay one step ahead in the treatment of sarcoidosis patients. An excellent concept!

When I asked Dan why he started Sarcoid Life, he told me this, "When someone is first diagnosed they need accurate, timely information. They need to be able to make well-informed decisions. When I was first diagnosed, I was told it will only last a few years, and that it was nothing to worry about. Well it's almost four years later, and it is definitely something to worry about. Most of all I formed Sarcoid Life to help people when they need it most. There are so many questions that arise after a diagnosis of sarcoidosis. Sarcoid Life can't answer them all, but I can try to help point them in the right direction. That's more than I had." Sarcoidosis non-profit organizations are written about later in this book.

You can contact Sarcoid Life by mail at **Sarcoid Life...4227 Peppermill Lane...Dallas, Texas 75287**. They also have an Internet website that can be accessed at **www.sarcoidlife.org** or either by way of the links page on my website, as addresses do change from time to time. A current phone number should be listed on the Sarcoid Life website.

As more people are diagnosed with sarcoidosis and with organizations like Sarcoid Life being created, hopefully positive results will come in the areas of finding the origin, testing and a cure for this disease. This is why it's important for stories such as Dan's and the rest of those in this book, are told. There is nothing to be ashamed of...You have a medical condition and after a while you start noticing common connections among the stories. By making people aware of patient stories and support organizations, awareness will increase and maybe in the future the patient or caregiver won't be the one who suggests looking for sarcoidosis. But until that time, keep advocating for yourself because once again, "It's your health that's at stake!"

3

MORE SARCOIDOSIS
VOICES

✦

E-mails From Sarcoidosis Patients

Over the past few years I've received e-mails from people who have either read my first book, read about my story on the Internet, read, heard or seen coverage of my story, or have visited my website. The e-mails have came from sarcoidosis patients, patients with other chronic health conditions, caregivers and those just interested in my story. They have been sent from all over the world. Some have been a call for help, while others just wanted to thank me for telling my story to help bring awareness to sarcoidosis, but most just wanted to tell their story to someone who could relate, as finding another sarcoidosis patient to talk to can at times, for a lot of patients, be difficult.

Although the stories were individually unique, they all had common grounds. The frustrations and past experiences all seemed to touch home in some form. I can honestly say each and every one of them touched my heart, so I wanted to share some excerpts from some of them with you, as I'm sure they will touch your hearts as well.

Unless noted, I do not know any of these people personally and have not even met them, although I've communicated with most of them online. I'm not going to include where they are from or their names and consequently can't personally verify that what they have written to me is true or accurate. But I can give you my word that the excerpts are as I received them and since I've heard the same types of experiences from many others, I have no reason to doubt their honesty. Unfortunately, I lost a lot of e-mails I had received about a year ago due to a computer crash, as they were saved on the hard drive. Since that time I've made backups on both my desktop and laptop…In today's computer environments, always make backups!

I want to start with a few excerpts regarding patients who have lived with sarcoidosis for a long time. Here's one from a gentleman who has had sarcoidosis for over 30 years. He wrote, ***"I can relate to your story as I was diagnosed with sarcoidosis in 1974. At the time I was into all types of sports, was married, and had three children. I became short winded, tired all the time, and being the big eater that I was, I couldn't keep food down. I had all the tests, and finally a lymph node diagnosis, and the doctors said "YOU HAVE SARCOIDOSIS". I said "Great, what is it, and is it curable?" They replied, "No, but we can treat the symptoms." I have been on prednisone, with a couple of short breaks, since I was diagnosed. I've been in and out the hospitals at least 15 times for kidney stones, stomach ulcers, hypocalcaemia, all the nails on my right hand turned ugly and brittle and I have blotches on my legs. My shortness of breath has hurt me in a lot of my daily activities and my job. Since my first experience I have come in contact with a few others that have it. I try not to let it get me down, when I find I can't do something I used to be able to do. I try it again and if I still can't I just don't. I am 55 yrs old and I have a lot of phobias and I know it's from being on the prednisone. I can tell you more but your probably dealing with it too. Be positive and don't let it win. I feel or have felt your pain"***

This excerpt is from a person whose grandmother had sarcoidosis and she thinks she might as well. She was giving me a history of her grandmother, ***"I'll start with my grandmother. The family moved to a farm up north in approximately 1909. She would have been about seven at the time. For grandma's diagnosis, it took three months and finally a biopsy to identify it in 1967 or 1968. Even major area medical centers were stumped. Grandma was of English decent. To her knowledge, 100% English. An interesting note about her siblings…All six of the children who reached adulthood had either heart or nervous system diseases or both. All the children at home in 1916 got diphtheria. The youngest died. The oldest later died of typhoid fever. One sister got extremely bad shingles on her legs. Their father died as a result of a cancerous brain tumor. Grandma's sarcoidosis was in her lymph nodes and did not go away. She struggled the remaining four years of her life with a constant battle between controlling the sarcoidosis with cortisone and her diabetes with insulin. She died due to a weakened heart, heart attacks and heart disease. She, like all her family, was stubborn and always kept going. She was active: planting, harvesting, canning, caring for her home (still hung laundry on the line to dry) and husband right up to a severe heart attack in October 1971. She died in 1972 at the age of 67."***

During my visits and speaking engagements at various sarcoidosis events, I found several people who are longtime sarcoidosis patients. This shows that sarcoidosis is not a new disease but has been around for a long time. In fact, Jonathan Hutchison, a surgeon-dermatologist at King's College in London, England, identified the first known case of sarcoidosis over a century ago. Since sarcoidosis is commonly misdiagnosed, especially in the past when it was often confused with tuberculosis, it makes you wonder how many people actually had sarcoidosis but never knew it. Just think how their lives would have been different if they were treated for the disease they actually had, not to mention probably lived a longer life. Although today we have gotten better at diagnosing patients with sarcoidosis, there is still a major need for more research and ways to detect the disease earlier.

Here's an e-mail that touched me in several ways, ***" I too have sarcoidosis and in my opinion I believe I've had it close to 20-25 years although I was diagnosed about seven years ago and at the time I was sure I was going to die. Today I'm living with it day by day. I'm finally off the prednisone after almost five years. I am now also diabetic. The added weight from cortisone therapy is resistant to dieting. My feet and hands hurt most of the time and keeps me from walking as much as I need to in order to lose some weight. Looking like Jabba the Hut is hard on the psyche! I'm having eyesight difficulties, but the doctors are not sure why. I see a local sarcoidosis specialist, which I located thru the Internet. My doctors at the time were going to handle it themselves until I had a drug reaction and they wouldn't take care of me and said to contact a dermatologist. So if they won't handle bumps and rashes I didn't want them taking care of my sarcoidosis. There are a lot of things I probably won't ever do again, but then again I'm still breathing. My goals are to see my kids get married and have kids themselves. I'm really trying hard to take care of myself. I once had a Neurologist tell me to divorce my husband and go on Medicaid so then at least the medical care wouldn't financially ruin my family. I do know that this is not "rare". I know of at least eight people thru people I know that have it. Sarcoidosis has to be pretty common but misdiagnosed as something else. Good thing I didn't settle on the lymphoma diagnosis!"*** How could any medical professional tell someone to get a divorce to save money on health care? Has the health care system in this country gotten that bad?

Here's another, ***"I read an interview you gave on sarcoidosis and it was great to see that you actually accomplished what I had planned to do for years, write a book on living with sarcoidosis. I tried but never finished, as my energy level or a part of me was always ill. Like you it took a long time for them to diagnose me with sarcoidosis. Some of the doctors I had seen made light of the disease and said it could go away without any more problems. I WISH! It has been nothing short of hell dealing with this disease! I have dealt with this for several years now. I lost at least a third of my lungs because of it, as I never regained the lost tissue. I had lumps of all kind and sorts on my body, some very large and others that I called purple measles. The strangest of all was that they got into my scars, which I have quite a few. It raised the scars and made them as hard as rocks and so painful. My glands, especially my parotid glands, swelled years ago and have never went down. Even my salivary glands no longer work. I guess you know all of this stuff I'm telling you, in fact I could go on and on with all the things I've experienced…The pain, nausea, sinus problems, sore throats, bowel problems as it's a never ending cycle. I just wanted you to know that there are more people out here suffering like you Gil. Like you, my Faith keeps me going one day at a time. Thank you for writing the book!***

Yet another patient seeking help, ***"I'm a 39 yr. old married female and so grateful I found your book as I've been dealing with debilitating illness for about 16 months now after previously leading a very active life. I have been granted Social Security disability, but still have no official diagnosis. As you keep saying in your book—not knowing the cause of your illness can be brutal on a person, mentally and emotionally. I was a newlywed, only six months married when this disease stopped me in my tracks. I have been pretty much housebound since then. I've been through so many tests, most with normal results. I'm scheduled to have a full body gallium scan which I'm praying will yield some answers. After months of research on my own, I feel convinced that sarcoidosis is the root of my illness, but pathological evidence is lacking so far. I have two first cousins who also have the disease. I see a doctor at a University medical center who feels that sarcoidosis is a possible diagnosis for me. Some of the unusual symptoms you mention that I share are the two toned skin (my cheeks have circular patches about the size of a half dollar that are several shades lighter than other skin on my face), the nose bleeds, fatigue, sun sensitivity, nausea, constant nasal congestion, extreme thirst and clear urine, frequent urination, lack of sex drive, decreased appetite, etc. I also have many of the neurosarcoidosis symptoms like cognitive difficulties, balance problems, vision problems, tingling, numbness, vertigo and dizziness along with the standard joint/body pain. You've heard it all before, I'm sure so thank you for listening to me. It helps to vent to someone who understands!"***

One more to make a point, ***" Thank you for writing about your experiences with sarcoidosis. Only God kept you because man could not have gone through so much and remained sane. I feel the same about my experiences. There have been times when I thought I was going to loose my mind, but had to remember who was keeping me and that He would help me through any and everything. I suffered with crohn's disease for four years before having surgery to remove nine inches of my colon. The surgery was in 1998. I had been on prednisone for four years straight. I was happy when I did not have to take that drug again. Then in March of 2002 I was diagnosed with pulmonary sarcoidosis. I was not put on prednisone until February 2003. I am on 2MG per day now. It's an awful drug but what can I do?"***

There are two points that stand out in not only these excerpts but in most e-mails I receive. First, there are the many forms of frustrations patients feel during the diagnosis period. This is just one reason why I stress, once again, the need for standardized tests to be developed and performed on a routine basis to look for sarcoidosis. The time has come to use research funds effectively and stop the many reasons why we have a hard time diagnosing sarcoidosis without performing a biopsy. I'm a perfect example of how the diagnosis period of (in my case) approximately five years caused a multitude of life altering permanent chronic health conditions that could have been prevented if only I had been correctly diagnosed from the beginning or at the very least in a few months. The need for awareness, education and proactive mindsets in regard to sarcoidosis must be observed and practiced by current medical professionals. As a patient it's also necessary to advocate for yourself as others have and force your medical professionals to look for sarcoidosis. It's your health at stake so do what you have to do while the medical profession becomes up to date in regard to sarcoidosis detection and treatments, which brings me to my second point...Prednisone.

Prednisone is used for a multitude of reasons and health conditions. It's an inexpensive drug and does a lot of good for a lot of people, including myself. It's also a primary treatment for sarcoidosis. As I've said before, personally I'm blessed that prednisone doesn't really bother me, except for the additional weight and round face effect. Of course, in reality, it probably does cause other problems as it has been given as a reason for my vision problems, irregular heartbeat, constant muscle cramps and others, but all in all it does me more good than bad (I assume), plus I have so many other situations that all bind together. However as you've read, others aren't as fortunate.

Aside from the ever present mental effect from factors such as weight gain, increased appetite and mood swings, a lot of people have major problems with the drug. It has been suggested that it's a contributing factor to other diseases and developing health conditions. Some people just can't take the drug physically.

My mother, for example, can't take prednisone without breaking out causing her to have a dangerous reaction. Others feel all kinds of side effects such as nausea, vomiting, indigestion, headaches, insomnia, dizziness, swollen legs or feet, poor wound healing, decreased or blurred vision, fever, mood or emotional changes, various infections, muscle cramps, stomach or hip or shoulder pain, fatigue, thirstiness, irregular heartbeat, convulsions, skin rash, joint pain, hallucinations, confusion, excitement, darkened or lightened skin color and euphoria; to just name a few mentioned in the "Complete Guide To Prescription & Nonprescription Drugs 2003 Edition". The interesting part is that for each of the previously mentioned side effects the suggested course of action is to continue to take and call your doctor. The only side effects mentioned in which the instruction is to seek emergency treatment immediately are hives, rash, intense itching, faintness and swelling soon after a dose (anaphylaxis). So you see, prednisone can be a rough drug for a lot of patients! Maybe with increased research we can find an alternate, but yet still effective, way to treat sarcoidosis for those who can't tolerate prednisone.

Here is one that touched my heart. ***"I am 24 years old and last year around this time I was diagnosed with sarcoidosis. It began two years before when I began having different problems but doctors never had any answers. Then last year I started having breathing difficulties. Some times I would feel like I was going to pass out. My doctors told me I was under too much stress and I was suffering from depression. I knew that could not be because I was and still am an "Oh Well" type of person. What I mean is that I never let life's trials get to me to the point where I can say I'm suffering from stress and depression. Around this time last year I started getting worse. I started having eye vision problems. My eye doctor told me that it looks like a condition called sarcoidosis. He sent me for a test with my doctor who performed a lung biopsy. It came back positive for type I sarcoidosis. This was a very sad time in my life because a woman at my church had just passed away from sarcoidosis in which her lungs fell. Now a year later since I found out, I am so scared each day of my life. I know that I don't need to be scared but I have a three year old daughter that I am taking care of and lately I have been very sick; in fact I just got out of the hospital Monday. As all of us, I have good days and bad ones, but what hurts the most is that I feel like I'm living all alone. I need to be strong for my baby but sometimes I can't help but to look at her and think, "Will I be around to see her grow up?" When I saw a story about you on the news I just wanted to contact someone who understood. I have support from my mom, who happens to be a minister, but she doesn't live with the condition so it's hard for her to really know what I go through. Please help me understand this a little more. I want my life back! I'm only 24 and even though I know I should be positive I can't help but think my life is supposed to be just starting not ending."***

This e-mail touched me deeply because of her young age. It makes it even harder mentally to deal with the hard realities of living with a disease that's not only mysterious but you know will be with you for the rest of your life. Not to mention the added stress of knowing someone personally who died from sarcoidosis. Hell, this is hard for me to deal with and I'm "quite a bit" older than 24 and have been dealing with my situation since 1986. But, as I mentioned in First Thoughts, when you know someone personally who dies as a result of sarcoidosis it puts a new reality on your situation and is a very difficult thing to deal with mentally…For anyone! I can't even imagine how I would have handled dealing with sarcoidosis when I was 24 years old. To be honest, at that time in my life I barely handled my life as a healthy young man.

This one gives a positive outlook from an experienced patient that we can all learn from. ***"I commend you on your positive attitude in spite of all of your secondary conditions. I had been sailing along smoothly with my condition, but now it seems to be progressing. It has affected my heart, thyroid and blood pressure. I have hand tremors and the doctors don't know what's causing them. They say it is not from my thyroid, although they found an antigen in my blood work and a small nodule on my right thyroid. When I was first diagnosed with sarcoidosis in 1976, I asked the big question, "WHY ME"? I now have an answer to that question and it is, "Why not me?" We all have some limitations, some more than others, but that's our life sprinkled with our own special seasonings (challenges). I am sure there is a message and reason for our unique situations. What helps me the most is staying as busy as I can by helping others. I volunteer at the hospital and I find it very rewarding. Our stay here is temporary and I would like to leave a legacy of love, compassion and empathy. Thank you for sharing your story! I am sure it gives others the courage to go on, as it has me. Each day is brand new and I hope this new day of yours will bring you joy, but if it does not, you have another one waiting in escrow."*** That really sums it up. What a positive attitude from someone who must truly be a very special person to the many people he or she comes in contact with. I wish we could all be so positive!

Another common theme to the e-mails I receive is the statement "I didn't know there were others out there like me" or "I've never met anyone else with sarcoidosis". Yes we are out here, more than you might expect. Here is an excerpt that describes what I mean. ***" I recently finished reading your book and just wanted to let you know what an inspiration it has been for me. I was diagnosed with stage I sarcoidosis in October of 2001. Not to bore you with too many of the details, but I was in the process of moving in the summer of 2001 and was experiencing some shortness of breath issues. I went to my doctor the day before I moved and I went in for what I thought was going to be my last appointment with him and he informed me that the chest X-ray came back abnormal and he wanted to do a CAT scan. Well, since the moving truck was already half way filled, I took the CAT scan order and had it performed at a hospital in the city in which I was moving. My wife (fiancé at the time) knew a good friend that was a doctor and took up overseeing my care once I got settled in. Well, when the CAT scan came back, they confirmed enlarged lymph glands in my chest. The doctor/friend of my wife prepared me for the worse. He told me all of the possible diagnoses that it could be as well as emphasized that nine out of ten times when he sees this in people my age, it is Hodgkin's disease cancer. At that point he got me into a great Oncologist who did some blood work and ordered a needle biopsy. Good news was the blood work came back fine, which all but ruled out cancer. But he still wanted to do a biopsy. Well the needle biopsy didn't work so they had to do a bronchoschopy biopsy. Once that was completed, the pathology results came back that it was sarcoidosis. Luckily for me, this whole process took about two months—a lot less than your five plus years.

From there, I was referred to a Pulmonologist who has been treating me since then. He has been checking me every three months for the last year and I am happy to say that the lymph nodes have gone back to normal size and my breathing is back to normal. Overall, my life has been somewhat okay with the situation. I still have the ability to exercise and play sports, work full-time and overall, carry on a 'normal' life (I use that word loosely). But I do experience some of the symptoms you talk about on a consistent basis.

Now the bad part…For the past six months I have been dealing with some severe chest pains and stomach problems that, to say the least, have not been fun. I have had more CAT scans, stress echos, X-rays, IVPs, gastroscopes, steroid treatments, and the list goes on. Needless to say they cannot find anything wrong and they can't determine if it is even related to my sarcoid. While it has been frustrating, it has been comforting reading your book as I have gone along with this process because it has given me a grounding point to deal with this. You did a great job of getting a good understanding of your situation across to your readers. It is also good to know that there is someone out there that is going through the same thing as me!!! I completely know how you are feeling with dealing with insurance companies, doctors, hospitals, COBRA, prescriptions, etc. as I work in the healthcare industry as a financial consultant. I am also thankful to my wife, who found your book. Actually, even my Pulmonologist was surprised to hear there was a book out there about the topic.

Anyway, I know I have gabbed on for far too long, but knowing that you would be in town, I wouldn't mind getting a chance to talk to you and meet you if you would like to talk in more detail. After reading your book, it would also be nice to have someone to talk to who understands this situation from a firsthand experience. Just having a conversation in person would be extremely beneficial to me. Looking forward to hopefully having that opportunity."***

Actually, I did have the opportunity to have lunch with this gentleman and his wife (I try to always sit down one on one with any patient when the opportunity arises), as it was also very beneficial for me. In fact, after he returned to his office his wife was heading my way and we had an opportunity to have a nice conversation on the benefits of her support of him. As with myself having a supportive spouse is something that you can't really describe in regard to the benefits it has on your ability to handle your health situation, especially when you are dealing with a disease like sarcoidosis. Having sarcoidosis affects everything in your life on a daily basis and in turn your spouse's life as well. Believe me, it's not a cakewalk for the spouse either, as we can be hard to deal with but as a team, which is what marriage really is, the rewards last for a lifetime! Let me give you another example of the rewards of this kind of teamwork.

It Affects More Than Just Men…

This last excerpt reinforced for me that what I was experiencing was not just happening to me. The last hurdle I had to get over before I had the courage to open up my story to the world for all kinds of scrutiny was the fact I was going to have to tell very personal aspects of my life. Being a private person (in fact before my first book not even my parents knew everything I had experienced and still do) it was extremely hard for me to get over this hurdle, but I knew I had to in order to write my story from a patient's perspective and keep it based on reality. I made the decision to go for it for two reasons.

The first was that everything we experience from a physical and mental perspective affects our overall health situation. If I was going to leave something out because it might be embarrassing or others might think I was crazy, then I might as well not write my story, but instead write a novel. After all, if everything wasn't told, then it was basically fiction. Since I wanted to write the truth to help others who might be going through similar situations, either with sarcoidosis or some other chronic health condition, then I had to tell it all…There was no other choice!

The second was that I shouldn't be embarrassed about anything I've experienced or experience, either physically or mentally, based on a health condition. Of course, when it came to subjects such as sexual functions or my mental outlook at times, this is a lot easier said than done. Sexuality is a very personal issue and when you have problems, especially as a man, it hurts your male pride and you will do everything you can to keep it as quiet as you can. This is wrong! Fortunately, with new medications and known unexpected individuals such as Bob Dole and professional athletes who have a macho image coming out publicly and talking about male sexual issues, it's becoming more open, therefore hopefully giving more men courage to seek help with their doctors.

Sex, or sharing of physical affection, is an important part (not the most important but still important) to a healthy relationship between a husband and wife. I remember when I first saw commercials about drugs that helped with male sexual problems I thought they were stupid until one day I actually thought about it then realized that they hit the nail on the head. There were several, but each one would have a man either at a party or at work and everyone was asking him questions such as did you get a haircut, have you lost weight, new suit, did you get back from vacation, been working out, get a raise, etc.? All questions based on the fact that he was somehow carrying himself with more confidence and had a renewed look of happiness about himself. Another has a man in the backyard rediscovering the ability to throw a football through a tire and enjoying himself again with confidence. In reality, these situations are so true because a fulfilling sexual life with your spouse will make a major difference in your overall outlook on life and more dramatically a dysfunctional sexual relationship in which you are too embarrassed to seek help for will make your life miserable. I know firsthand, because before I was diagnosed with insufficient testosterone levels due to sarcoidosis being on my pituitary gland, it was a major issue for me mentally. Fortunately, I had a very supportive girlfriend, who became my wife, as we built our relationship not on sex but on mutual respect for each other. Without her I would have been in trouble mentally as this is something you don't openly discuss with the fellows. But it's not just male issues, as females experience the same frustrations. After all, sharing sex does take two!

One of the most frequent complaints I hear from women on prednisone is the issue of weight gain and what it does to their confidence and self-esteem. "How can I feel attractive with all of this added weight?" they will ask. Part of lovemaking is the mental aspect that you feel attractive and sexy in order to turn on your partner. This goes both ways but is especially important for women. There is so much more to lovemaking than just intercourse!

In addition, when you are not feeling well, tired or just can't seem to function, making love is not on the top of your list and if you had a date planned with your partner the mental aspect that you feel you let them down adds to the frustrations, even if your partner is understanding and provides no pressure. This is a normal human emotion.

So, not only will the man feel more confident with a good sex life, the woman will as well. Don't be embarrassed! Seek help because you have a medical condition. By no means does it make you any less of a man or woman. Understand what you are dealing with…Honestly accept it…Then get help so you can get back to a normal life!

I actually met this woman in person while speaking at a sarcoidosis event and spoke with her briefly as she bought one of my books. She was in her 40s and was on constant oxygen due to the fact that one of her lungs was nonfunctional due to sarcoidosis. A few days later she wrote, ***" I welcomed the open and honesty of your book as it pertains to sexual dysfunction. Sexual dysfunction as a result of medication, chronic illness, etc. is a subject I wish we could be more open about. Thanks for opening the door to that very real problem that needs discussing. Sexual activity is very strenuous and I thought I would stop breathing if I had intercourse with my husband. So instead I tried to avoid it. He became frustrated and then I became frustrated. Plus I felt unattractive with having a cannoli up my nose giving me oxygen during intimacy. How attractive is that? I overcame it by going deep within my soul and asked, "Do you want to look attractive during intercourse or do you want to be able to breathe and enjoy yourself?" Well, the latter won! The first time my husband asked, "Do you want me to get your oxygen?" before one of our intimate moments I knew that we'd reached a higher level of acceptance, love and understanding. Right today he doesn't know how unattractive I felt with that tube up my nose during intimate moments…Or maybe he does. But now it's no big deal and what a difference it made in our lives once we were able to accept my situation as it is. There are a lot of people dying to talk about this but are too embarrassed. Thanks for sharing that most private part of your life."*** Always remember…Don't be embarrassed about what you feel physically or mentally and most importantly seek medical help. It's your health and quality of life at stake!

I could go on with examples as I've received so many other touching e-mails outside of these. A lot ask for information regarding support groups so they can talk to someone who might understand what they are experiencing. Some are from caregivers who want to know what they can do to help their loved ones, as their loved ones shut them out. I can't say it enough...Open honest communication is the key for all parties. The frustrations are on both parties so be honest about what you feel and more importantly listen to what others in your life tell you. Listening is an important skill in building relationships of any kind. There are other e-mails from individuals just wanting to vent their stories, as they have no one in their lives that understand or take the time to just listen to them.

Others want advice on how to deal with others at work. They feel their employers and co-workers do not understand or care about what they experience. This creates an isolation between the patient and those in their work lives that not only causes additional frustrations and mental stress on all parties but is also from a business standpoint nonproductive and at times outright illegal. There is no reason a person with sarcoidosis can't be productive. Maybe not in the same manner they were before their diagnosis, but why throw away a valuable employee with years of positive experience when, with minor adjustments, you could keep that expertise? As a businessman, that just makes logical ethical business sense to me. Unfortunately though, in reality, that's not how it always is. This is one reason for a need to have the Americans with Disability Act (ADA) that requires employers to make reasonable adjustments to employ workers with disabilities or who might need special assistance, as long as it doesn't hurt the business. There are a lot of success stories, but in the same tone, all business people don't comply. Stand up for your rights if you are in that situation and research your rights. This is your quality of life we are talking about so stand firm!

I welcome all e-mails in the future as I personally open, read and reply to them in a usually timely manner, unless I'm unavailable for some reason or behind in my replies. Your honest e-mails inspire me and help me just as much as it might help you to get things off your chest. You can always reach me via my website and you are never bothering me (this is a common sentence on most of the e-mails). Communication is a two-way street and I need communication with others who can relate to my situation as much as you need communication with someone who can relate to yours. So thank you to anyone who has ever sent me an e-mail!

"Excerpts from e-mails are included between the quotation mark/three asterisks"

4

CHILDREN & SARCOIDOSIS

✦

They Too Are Part Of The Equation

Our children are our future! This is an important statement to remember. As parents and adults we are responsible for the upbringing of our children. The values they develop are based on what we teach them and the environment we set for them to learn about life. As adults we are a reflection of our parents and the adults we were exposed to as children. From them we learned our values and how to overcome or deal with our environments and life situations we encounter on a daily basis. This chapter is about our children, because everything we do reflects on them and just because a parent or adult has sarcoidosis or a child has the disease, doesn't change this fact of life.

First, let me stress that I'm not a Child Psychiatrist or a Pediatrician. I was raised an only child in North Florida in the 1960s and 1970s. My mother was an elementary school teacher and my father was a high school teacher, along with being a basketball coach, football coach and softball umpire (a big deal in North Florida). I grew up in a very diverse environment, around different cultures and environments, even though I was raised in the rural South. I easily adapted to the adults in my life and also to the street environment for which I spent a majority of my personal time. Being a very good basketball player I spent a lot of time on the playgrounds and in the gyms. As an only child I also learned how to adapt to being alone. I learned from all of these environments, but most importantly I always listened to the older folks, as they would teach me about life. This is one thing in America we seem to lack and that's the respect for older Americans. There's a lot of wisdom we can obtain from their experiences; both from the positive things they have done and the mistakes they are willing to teach us not to make ourselves. How many times have you heard people say, including yourself, "If I could only start over knowing what I know now?" Well, if you had listened to the adults in your life at the time, maybe you could have known more than you did and therefore not made some of the mistakes you did. There is also a tendency not to listen to the younger generation as well. But the reality is they too have feelings, ideas and a fresh wisdom that if we listened to, we might actually learn something. Our older generation and our younger generation make us who we are.

When I decided to write about other patient's stories I wanted to include a story about children with sarcoidosis, as they too suffer from the disease. As a child it can be even more difficult dealing with a chronic health condition, especially one like sarcoidosis. Your body is constantly changing causing your symptoms to change as well. The many visits to doctors, both before and after diagnosis, would wear you down, along with giving you the feeling of not being normal, as the other kids don't have to go through what you do. But the real battle, I would think, would be mental. It's difficult for adults to handle the mental aspect of sarcoidosis and the physical limitations it can impose on you, but for a child it can have an even more dramatic effect. I can't even imagine going through my childhood dealing with the health issues I've dealt with since 1986. Even if that's all you know in your young life, just watching the other kids would give you a lonely feeling, as you are left out of many normal childhood activities. Then there is the fact of life that children are innocent and haven't learned the phoniness of being tactful or not saying what's on their mind, when it's on their minds…In other words children can be brutally cold to other children, especially those children that are deemed "different".

"They" say sarcoidosis is rare among children, but then "they" also say it's a rare disease period, so take that statement for what it's worth…Not much in my opinion. Children patients too must go through the many tests and doctors visits, just as adult patients do. But a major difference is that the results are not discussed with the child patient, but instead they are discussed with the parents or adult who takes care of the child. Now this is understandable, but for a second imagine if you had to endure test after test, feeling the way you do and the doctors only look at you and smile, while discussing your health with someone else. You have no idea what is going on except that you feel bad and can't play like the other kids do. This has got to be a mental stress that I know, from a personal standpoint, I can't relate to.

As a child you are not yet prepared to do extensive research or understand the medical terminology being thrown around you, but never directly to you. You don't even know your body the way an adult should know theirs, as a child's body continues to grow and change. As an adult the lack of information and understanding regarding sarcoidosis is overwhelming at times, so for a child you can only imagine the feelings they encounter. After all, they are human too and the need to understand what you are feeling is a basic human feeling.

Then there are the parents. It's hard enough for a caregiver to be a spouse and in a lot of cases a spouse can't take the pressure, therefore the relationship breaks up. But with your child you can't just end the relationship and walk away. This isn't someone you chose to be with, this is part of your body, soul and blood. You created this person, so the hurt a parent must feel is something again, I can't relate to. It tore me up inside to see my stepdaughter get hurt in normal ways while growing up, so I have no idea how I could handle it if she had to take the journey of living with sarcoidosis. Would I feel guilty or somehow responsible? Would I be able to handle the emotional aspect of seeing her go through all of the necessary tests with uncertain results? Would I be able to look her in the eyes and explain honestly to her what was going on with her health wise? Would I be able to handle the financial responsibility of dealing with all of the medical expenses, along with the everyday expenses of raising a child? Would I be able to discipline her when she did something wrong, knowing all the pain she must be in? Would I even feel at times comfortable around her? The truth is…I don't know. However, I do know that I would always ask God each and every day to let me take her place. These are just a sample of what a parent whose child suffers from sarcoidosis experiences, on top of their own responsibilities and problems.

But the fact is children do get sarcoidosis and other chronic health conditions. Like adults, although all cases are different based on the disease, there are so many similarities. Since I can't honestly communicate what it's like to raise a child with sarcoidosis, I asked a parent, who could, if she would tell us her story of raising a daughter battling sarcoidosis. She agreed.

Now the story you are about to read was uniquely conducted in comparison to the previous or future stories in this book, for a couple of reasons. First, as you know, it's my policy to only write patient stories as the patient tells them to me personally, because only the patient truly knows how they feel. Well, it's the mother of the child who suffers from sarcoidosis, as I have never spoken to the child directly, that tells this story to me. It would be unfair and against my principle to put the child through the interview process directly, as she experiences enough. Plus do you remember the details of your health situation when you were one year old? I don't. So please keep that fact in mind.

Secondly, nowhere in the story or in this book, will I mention anything that will connect you to the child. There is no way I would ever put a child though the labeling of a sarcoidosis patient, or any adult for that matter, without their permission, and to be blunt, a child of this age just can't make that decision. Therefore, I will not mention her name, except to say that she is female, her parents name or her living environment, except to say she lives in the United States. There will be no nicknames such as Baby Jane or Baby X, as this is a real child who deserves more respect than to be labeled a nickname. This isn't a game or hyped up fiction story, this is reality that affects a…Real…Living…Innocent…Child. We must always keep that in perspective.

In addition, there will be no mention of her or her family in the "Acknowledgment Section" of this book, so let me say now, "Thank You" to the family for providing this story and giving me permission to use it in this book. I know, without a doubt, it will touch many hearts and make many people think about sarcoidosis, because as I've said many times over…Sarcoidosis can affect any organ or gland in the body, including the eyes, skin and spine…Sarcoidosis can affect anyone regardless of race, sex, age, financial status, living environment, sense of humor or any other factor you want to include…Sarcoidosis truly shows no prejudice! Here is a perfect example of what those statements mean.

A Child's Story…

The time was November 1998. A father and mother were looking at their beautiful, healthy, newly born daughter for the first time. It was their second child, the other being a boy, just a few years older. Their lives quickly transformed to adjusting to a newborn. For the first six months everything was "normal", if you can call having a newborn around the house "normal". When you have a newborn everything, and I mean everything, in your life changes. Just going to the corner store becomes an adventure. But no one in this happy family was complaining.

In May 1999, the newborn went for her routine six months check-up. The examination resulted in healthy reports and of course, vaccinations. She received the standard vaccinations, along with the first dose of a four part series of rotashield vaccines. At the time, rotavirus had been the cause of an increased number of children being hospitalized and this vaccine was highly recommended. As the mother tells me, "I continuously go back to this date because, in my opinion, this was the beginning of our journey with sarcoidosis."

After the series of vaccines, the newborn started to develop a hive reaction. When the doctor took a look at the rash, she confirmed that the baby was having some type of negative reaction. Okay, this is fairly normal, even with adults when they are given some type of medication for the first time. No need for alarm...Until.

One night in July 1999, the mother was sitting with her newborn watching the nightly newscast. A story came on the broadcast that not only got her immediate attention, but also changed her, and her daughter's life, forever. Rotashield had been taken off the market! The mother recalls asking herself in a panic frame of mind, as her heart landed in her stomach, "What had I done to my baby?" A mother's worst nightmare was just beginning.

The hive reaction did not go away, in fact it continued, changing appearances from day to day and spread all over her tiny body. Her mother described it by saying, "It got to the point I was almost afraid of what the rash was going to look like from one day to the next. I can clearly remember dropping down on my knees sobbing each morning, as I would find this "thing" overcoming my beautiful baby's body. I felt helpless."

From May 1999 to October 1999, the parents took the baby from doctor to doctor, clinic to clinic and hospital to hospital. They saw Pediatricians, Dermatologists and Ophthalmologists, searching for anyone to come up with an answer, or better yet, a cure for this rash taking over their child's life. They tried everything they could think of, such as treating the child for eczema, using topical cream after topical cream, greasing her down with lotions, but still the rash seemed to have a mind of its own, as it continued to go as it pleased. The lack of answers devastated the parents, not to mention the cruel stares and rude comments strangers would make when the family was out in public. We as human beings can be so cold to our fellow human beings, especially when we don't have a clue as to what the other people are experiencing. If only we would treat our fellow human beings as we would like to be treated ourselves, every second of every day. Just think how much better this world would be? But we all know that's not the case and no matter how hopeful or positive you might be, it never will be that way, so let's move on.

The baby was seen at a local university medical center, as the doctors and students alike gathered around her like she was a freak show. The child was pricked, poked, photographed, examined and studied so many times that the parents lost count. By this time the rash had literally covered her from head to toe and the only explanation they ever got from any of the specialists, doctors or students was, "You have a beautiful, healthy little girl, who happens to have a rash. It'll clear up soon." Well, this was unacceptable, so off to check for an infectious disease and try that route, but still no diagnosis...Only puzzlement.

Her hands and feet now had raised pink bumps covering them. Her face and the rest of her body were covered with tiny pin dot rashes that began to invade the whites of her eyes as well. Her mother recalls, "Her eyes turned pink in color and resembled a gritty texture like chewing gum rolled in sand." She often became photosensitive, turning beat red very quickly, resembling sunburn. Although you can only imagine what a child of that young age is feeling, she looked very uncomfortable and at times her arms, feet and face appeared to be swollen. As a helpless mother's heart went out to her child she says, "My little one had endured so much in her few months of life and yet remained a real trooper."

In October 1999, they were finally able to get into a nationally known clinic, but what an overwhelming and exhausting experience that turned out to be. They spent most of their time going through multiple examinations, blood tests and skin biopsies, with an Ophthalmologist and Dermatologist, to determine "what" was wrong with their child. By this time the parents felt numb to the physical aspect from this seemingly forever journey, but from a mental aspect, they were reaching their limits, as they desperately prayed for answers, while at the same time, scared to death of the unknown. That evening, after a full day at the clinic, they received a call from the Dermatologist at 10:00 PM. The mother can still hear the voice in her head today, as it said, "I need to see you back here first thing in the morning. I believe your daughter has sarcoidosis."

Immediately a thousand questions ran through her mind…"What?"…"What is sarcoidosis?"…"How?"…"What did I do wrong?"…"Why?"…"Will it go away?"…"What do we do?"…"Will she die?"…And so on and so on, as she and her husband personally dealt with the fact that their daughter had just been diagnosed with something neither had ever even heard of. The doctors were just as amazed, as they had never seen sarcoidosis in a child so young. The next morning resulted in more tests, as the baby was started on heavy doses of prednisolone, to try to drown out the fire that was burning within her young body. The positive news was that she responded well to the medication, as finally her skin started to clear up.

She has had to be put under anesthesia multiple times so that the Ophthalmologist could perform eye biopsies, take pictures of her eyes and monitor her condition. Although granulomas were found in the back of her eye, her vision, as of yet, has not been affected. In addition to her eyes, sarcoidosis has affected her skin. The good news is that it hasn't spread to any other organs in her tiny body. That's a small miracle in itself!

The clinic staff has become like family and the positive part is that the family is satisfied with the care they have received. This is a major plus and the kind of thing I personally love to hear. It's a good thing too, because they return to the clinic on a regular basis. Each month, and sometimes more frequently, they return to monitor the child's condition with blood tests, eye examinations and vision tests. There are also very specific annual exams and testing that occurs.

There is also the constant medications required, some of which she has had negative reactions to. However, when the medications are decreased or stopped, there is an instant increase in the inflammation in the child's eyes and the rash reappears. In addition, the child has developed an ulcer, so now not only are there eye and skin concerns, but also there is an abundance of "tummy" complaints, and the ever present pain the child must endure. This tears the mother's heart apart, as it would any mother who had to watch so much medication dumped into their little girl's body, along with watching the constant pain that has become a "normal" part of her young life.

Just to give you an idea of this young girl's medication routine, at this time in her life, she is required to take prednisolone eye drops six times a day, systemic prednisolone every other day, carafate three times per day for the ulcer, miralax once a day to care for the constipation that carafate causes, a weekly injection of methotrexate and has recently been introduced to enbrel, which is another series of injections twice a week. All of this, just to maintain the inflammation that burns through her young body as a result of sarcoidosis. And to think, we thought we had it bad!

All things considered, her mother describes her as a "model patient". The drawing of blood, IV's and injections are the toughest part for her, as her mother puts it, "She hates the needle thing, as it's always somewhat of a struggle." Trust me…This I can relate to, as I hate needles! Periodically, she will have spells in which she can become very dehydrated and lethargic very quickly. No one is sure exactly what this is or why. She may be over-stimulated, as her body does not digest her food properly and instantly shuts down. She'll start vomiting and basically be completely wiped out. Sometimes the mother can catch it and treat her with pedialyte popsicles, other times, it's off to the emergency room for an IV. These spells can impact her for a day, or it can wipe her out for days on end, and have now just become another of the many uncertainties that are a part of everyone's life.

As the child becomes of school age, another fear has surfaced…What will she be able to tolerate and what will she be exposed to? For example, she can't have a chicken pox vaccine, or any other live vaccines for that matter. If she is exposed to someone, face-to-face, for as little as five minutes, who has been exposed or has chicken pox themselves, the mother has 72 hours to get her to the hospital for a

VZIG transfusion. The results of her getting chicken pox would be extremely serious, requiring hospitalization at the least, or worse. So this is serious stuff, as kids come to school with all kinds of things…Pink eye comes to mind as well, which are very contagious.

Needless to say, the family has become, as the mother states, "We are complete germ freaks. We have our own routine when we use public restrooms and about what we all touch when in public. We are continuously washing our hands throughout the day, whether we're in public or at home. Germs are always on our minds." They also make sure the school nurse is aware of the seriousness of this situation. In fact, she will call the mother if a chicken pox case is reported at her older brother's school. Open, honest communication is such a powerful tool and this family doesn't hesitate to use it in every aspect of their lives.

But even with all of the physical challenges and medications required, we as sarcoidosis patients know the hardest part is mental. This situation is no different, but in fact, is more involved, as we now not only have a young patient, but also the caregivers are parents, with unique feelings and responsibilities other than "normal" caregivers.

Up until around four years old or so, all that this young child was experiencing was "normal" to her. After all, she had been going through all of these experiences since she was less than a year old. This was all she knew. So how was she to know this was not "normal"? But around this time she started asking questions to her parents, as she was exposed to more in life than just her immediate home and medical facilities.

There were questions like…"Why do I have to go to the doctor so much?"…"Why do I need so much medication?"…"Why do I have to get so many shots?"…"Why can't I play like the other kids?"…"Why doesn't my brother have to do all of this?"…"Am I normal?"…Well, you get the picture. I can't even begin to imagine the mental outlook of this child, and to be honest; no one else can either, including her parents or medical professionals. But by the questions she asks, you can get some idea of what must be going through her developing mind. After all, this is a child, with a child's mind that is growing everyday, as she is exposed to the newness of life itself, but yet dealing with health issues that an adult would find hard to deal with without going crazy or falling into a deep state of depression. Maybe being a child is an advantage, because what else does she know? I don't have a clue! However I can say, just by what I know about this case, this young girl has a strong mind and my utmost respect…That's for sure!

Now from a caregiver or parent's perspective, although once again I can't personally relate, we can get an idea, based on the questions the mother ponders, of what a mother goes through in these types of situations, from a mental perspective. She asks herself questions such as…"Why can't anyone tell me what will tomorrow bring?"…"Why is sarcoidosis always labeled as a mysterious disease?"…"Will sarcoidosis ever leave my daughter's body?"…"Why and how did she get it, as there is no family history of sarcoidosis?"…"How could a child six months old get a disease that commonly affects people 20+ years old?"…"What invaded her immune system?"…"Was it something in the environment or something I did?"…"Will she be on medication all her life?"…"Will the sarcoidosis one day affect or take her vision?"…"Will she be able to have children of her own one day and if so will they have sarcoidosis?"…"What research is being done for sarcoidosis and will they find a cure during my daughter's lifetime?"…"How is information being distributed to the sarcoidosis community so if a positive treatment is found, how will my daughter benefit?"…"Will she ever be able to enjoy just one carefree day at the beach, as a normal teenager?"…"Will she make it to the prom?"…There are so many questions and absolutely no concrete answers.

The most frustrating part is the unknown and it's something the family must always deal with. The mother went on to say, "I felt horrible and felt that I had to explain to everyone, as people would look at my daughter then look at me when we were out in public. I never knew how she was going to look from one day to the next. I'd break down in tears in the morning when I'd go pick her up out of her crib. At the end of the day, I never knew what I was going to see when I picked her up from daycare…It was really tough. I wasn't sleeping, therefore I was constantly exhausted. I dropped weight instantly and just felt like I was going through the motions. I remember the day she was diagnosed. I sat up on the couch all night and cried and cried. This was just something that I had to do, before I could accept the news we had received. I guess everyone needs a "woe in me" moment. As far as how have I mentally handled all of this? We have good days and bad days. When she seems status quo, life is good. Otherwise, I just deal with the moment the best way I can."

She continued by adding, "A medical calendar was a necessity, just to keep track of what medications were needed and when, as well as how my daughter was feeling, and the on-going state of her condition. I document everything! This has been a godsend to me and the other caregivers/doctors, as we reference back through time to compare what has worked, what has not, what progress has been made, and what setbacks we've had. This calendar helps keep me current and on track, as I remain the strongest advocate for my daughter. I've learned to ask lots of questions, and to continue to press further when I'm unsatisfied with an answer. I also found great relief in keeping a journal of our experiences. My daughter will have very interesting reading one day."

Well, for whatever it's worth, one question I can answer for her and her husband is, without a doubt, based on everything I know about this case, "NO" you as parents did nothing wrong! In fact, you both have done everything possible to find what was causing your daughter's health problems and supported her unconditionally. The mental stress for parents in these types of situations, not to even get into the financial burdens, where you did everything right, then the unexpected comes along, can be overwhelming, to say the least. This is when you need support more than can be described. Fortunately, this family does have outlets.

Aside from the positive relationships they have built with their medical professionals, they also have support from other family members, including the older brother. The mother describes the son like this, "From a sibling perspective, I am fortunate to have a son with a very, very kind and emotional heart. He is very protective of his sister and also deals with all that we must undergo." However, we must remember that he is a child as well. At times he gets frustrated by all of the attention his sister receives. Obviously, when she is having a bad day it impacts the entire family and any activities that might have been planned. When those times come up, the father tries to spend more time with his son and give him the fatherly attention that is critical to his development, as the mother takes care of the daughter.

In regard to the other family members, everyone has been very supportive. They ask questions on her status, listen and offer thoughts that the parents, or the doctors, may not have thought of or brought up. She told me, "In the early stages, my sister started out reading everything she could on the Internet, trying to educate herself. Some things she would pass along, others she would not because she didn't want to upset or scare me. Our family helps the most by just being there to listen. That's what I need, they let me talk and offer suggestions. They call to check on us all the time and await the news from every doctor visit. From a Faith perspective, my daughter is always in my family's prayers." In addition, the daughter goes to the family day care and is looked after by family members, which has been wonderful for support, as they administer the medications and help keep detailed track of everything that goes on. This is a real team effort and is a perfect example of how a family should come together, sharing responsibilities and just being available, so that everyone benefits.

Her teachers have also been on top of the situation, although it can be difficult. After all, even though they are fully aware of the situation, they also have other kids who need equal attention. They too ask themselves questions such as…"Are we treating her the same as everyone else?"…"What are we creating with all of this attention?"…"Are we giving too much attention and hurting the process of her learning on her own?"…"How do we know when or if we are over-compensating?"…"Are we building resentment from the other kids, therefore creating an environment where she can never be a normal child?"…Again, you get the picture. Good teachers are a special breed of people who love their profes-sion…I know because both of my parents were excellent teachers who taught for the love of teaching. Let's just pray all of her teachers are special because teachers have a major impact on our children. Having sarcoidosis doesn't change that fact.

Another major positive support outlet has been the mother's employer, actu-ally two of them. She explains, "In the initial stages of trying to get my daughter diagnosed, I was out of the office a lot. I had an unbelievable employer who con-sistently told me, "It's okay; you need to do what you need to do." He never questioned my time outside the office and was very supportive. I was later approached by another company, and actually changed employers. As part of my interview process, I was very open from the start as to what my daughter's condi-tion was and could mean. Since that timeframe, they too have been supportive. I've been fortunate that she has had very minimal consecutive days in which I've had to be away from work. Most of our clinic appointments, which are monthly, we leave around five in the morning to get an early doctor visit so that I can get back to work at a decent time, as the clinic is an hour and a half drive away from our home. Most times for regular appointments, I try to schedule them after work hours, if I can. In addition, I work from home after hours to catch up, when needed, to make sure my office responsibilities do not slip. Overall I've had nothing but positive results and support."

Now let me say a couple of things about what she just said to make a point that I've been talking about for ages. First, always be honest with your employer upfront. A lot of people look at me like I'm crazy when I say this but the bottom line is if you have a chronic health condition to deal with then the time is going to come when you have to deal with it, whether you are a patient or caregiver. If your employer can't handle it upfront then they surely aren't going to be able to handle it when it affects your work schedule. Honesty and understanding about what you are dealing with upfront goes a long way, especially in the business world. Secondly, your employer owes you nothing…You owe each other. You should do work on your own and go out of your way to ensure your job responsi-bilities are covered. This is what business is about…Meeting the requirements and bottom line. Your relationship is a team effort and you both must make adjustments in order to succeed. If you do then you both will be successful, which again is the ultimate goal. You don't think it makes a difference? Then reread the previous paragraph!

I must admit, although this story was personally hard for me to write from an emotional standpoint, there are some positive points that touched me. For one is the support of the family. A perfect example of coming together in times of need, as opposed to just at family gatherings when everyone is there primarily for a good meal. Another is the positive support of their medical professionals, again something that is critical and good to see. Then there is the support of the teachers and others who interact with this child. Last is the support of the employers in handling this special situation and getting positive results by caring about their employee and vice versa. Regardless of all the negatives I hear regarding these points, especially in regard to sarcoidosis patients, this shows that positives really can take place, if only people are honest and put forth the effort. My hat is off to all of those involved…You know who you are!

My prayers are also with this lovely little girl and her family, as they still have a journey ahead of them. But there are also many other families and little girls and boys out there who must deal with sarcoidosis. This is just one story of many. If all of the other reasons why we need to increase awareness regarding sarcoidosis and start taking research seriously, such as who is going to get the funding, political issues or whatever other reasons/excuses keep us from moving on, do not appeal to you, then do it for the children…Present and future. We've got to come up with answers, as I personally never want to write another story such as this one. And if you still can't feel the urgency to promote sarcoidosis awareness and fund research then ask yourself this, "What if it was my child?" I bet that would make a difference in your train of thought!

We As Sarcoidosis Adults…

Another situation regarding children, that I have experience with and can relate to, is the effect we adults who have sarcoidosis or any other chronic health condition have on the children in our lives. As I've stated many times, having a chronic health condition affects everyone in your life, including your children. As adults with the responsibility of raising our children (not just our own but also those you have daily contact with and influence over) we must ensure we do not negatively impact those children because of our health issues. Let me explain what I mean by this.

One of the beauties of children is the fact you can treat them almost any kind of way and they will forgive you. For example, if you miss an important date with them they will forgive you almost as soon as they see you. This is one of the pure joys of being a child…Innocents and the ability to unconditionally forgive in hopes that next time will be different. But after time and the next times never changes, even a child will start to have doubts. The bad part about this is that the child will most likely think the reason you don't show up is because of them…It's somehow their fault. You can't let this happen because the unjust negative impact on that child can last a lifetime.

This is why you must be honest with your children about your health condition. They must understand to the best of their ability that you have a health condition that keeps you from doing certain things in life that you would love to do, such as being able to attend that date you missed. They must understand to the best of their ability that your health kept you from attending and it had absolutely nothing to do with the child. They did nothing wrong!

That repeated term "honest open communication" with your children is the key to developing a lifelong relationship and positive self-esteem for your children. How you tell them will depend on several factors such as their age, maturity level, emotional state of being, along with other basic factors that make us all unique. So you must determine how much you want to tell them without confusing them, which will lead to frustration on their part and possibly blaming themselves anyway. As adults we know how complicated sarcoidosis can be, so try these methods.

First, teach them how to pronounce sarcoidosis. If they can pronounce the word then it might not seem so mysterious to them. Try to keep it simple and on their level, increasing the information as they get older. Explain to them how it makes you feel as opposed to exactly what it is. For example "Sarcoidosis is in my body and makes me feel real tired a lot of times, like how you feel after you have been playing or just before you go to bed. Sometimes it makes me feel sick, like when you have a bad cold and have to miss a day of school. I take medicine to help me but there are some times when I just can't do things I really want to do, like do the things I love doing with you. I hope you will understand it has nothing to do with you but it's my health that keeps me from doing things with you at times. But when those times happen, as soon as I feel better we can do something you want to do, you just tell me what because I love you and love doing things with you." Always try to include an example of something in their lives so they can have something to relate what you are saying back to something they understand. Repeated conversations such as this will instill the fact in your child's mind that you have a health condition and it has nothing to do with them.

Also, help them feel involved with your health. If they want to bring you some water then let them, then tell them how much help they are. Acknowledge when they clean their room or maybe wash the dishes by telling them what a positive difference it makes when they help you out. This will not only give them self-esteem but will teach them responsibility, two positive traits children need to learn from their parents.

Another important point you need to make sure you teach them is, for one, how to dial 911. This might seem simple but if you are not able to communicate then they need to know how to call for emergency help, know their address and how to communicate this information over the phone. In addition they need to know where you keep your medical information that includes details of your health condition, medications, insurance information and emergency contacts. Have it somewhere easy to find because it could be your children will be the only people available to save your life. Make sure they are aware and prepared! Like fire drills, it doesn't hurt to practice.

But the most important thing you can do is simply keeping your word to them. Always follow up on what you tell them you will do and if for some reason (and there will be those times in life) that you are not going to be able to follow up, make sure you tell them as soon as you know, and tell them the truth. The most important thing you can do is whenever you are feeling better use that time to spend with your children. Your time and attention is what they really want! If you don't feel like getting out, because keeping up with children can be very tiring, sit down with them, turn off the television or video games and read together or just talk. Let them lead the conversation and talk about what they want to, as you become a good listener then give them the benefit of your wisdom. Remember, this is their time with you as opposed to your time with them. Answer any questions they might ask you about not only your health but also life in general and please answer them honestly, giving as many details as you can based on their age. Always find an opportunity to teach, because it's from you that they learn the basic values of life. Don't just answer their questions, but when possible explain to them "why" it is like it is. As a parent you are laying the foundation of values for their life so teach them the truth, because they are going to learn the truth one day anyway, so what better person to learn it from than the adults in their lives whom they trust?

It's also healthy for your children to see you as a human being, just like them. You make mistakes, have emotions and must deal with problems the same as them. A lot of parents want to "protect" their children from real life situations, such as health problems, by keeping everything from them and putting them in a bubble. What does this help? How are they going to react when they have never seen nor experienced failure or problems of their own nor have they even seen their parents dealing with life's issues? An educated guess would be, not very good! I know it's hard to tell your children about unpleasant situations, such as your health, because you don't want them to worry or worse yet watch them make mistakes or fail. But it's a fact of life that they are going to experience these situations, so why not teach them how to deal with worrying, mistakes and failure as a child so that by the teenage years, when there will be a lot of worrying, mistakes and failures, along with peer pressure, they are prepared? Protecting them only sets them up to be taught by who knows who. Do you really want the local tough guy or the girl who thinks she knows it all teaching your child the facts of life and their values? It might seem like they aren't listening, but in reality they are storing that information you teach them in their memory banks and when the time comes it will pop into their main memory. However, if you never teach them then their memory banks will be blank and the negative influence will have no knowledge or logic to overcome what their "not so smart" peers are telling them.

I was always taught that if you don't make mistakes then you aren't doing anything in your life. No mistake is a mistake, the first time. There is nothing to fear in failure but you have everything to fear by not trying. Wondering "what if" is the worst thought you can have to live with. Teach your children not to be afraid to try, just as you are not afraid to deal with your health situation openly. Lead by example. Show them that just because you are having a bad day today, tomorrow will be better, because you will make it better, and if not, then you will try harder the next day. Life is not easy, so please don't build a false world around your children because eventually they will have to live in the same world as everyone else. Make sure they are prepared! That's your responsibility as a parent and just because you have sarcoidosis or some other chronic health condition doesn't excuse you from that responsibility nor does it keep you from teaching your children the correct values in life.

Don't fool yourself into thinking you can hide your health issues from your children. They see you every day and aren't stupid. In fact, children have a remarkable sense for how adults around them feel. We as adults should give them more credit. If the truth were known, maybe we are the ones who are clueless most of the time, not our children. They watch your every move and learn from what you do and say, whether you are intentionally teaching them or not, so be aware. Be honest with them and most importantly…Spend time with them every chance you get. Even if you can't get out of bed on this day, welcome them to your room and just talk. Don't shut them out just because your ego doesn't want them to see you like this. They need you and you are who you are, life is what it is. Always have time for your children because they are our future and our future is in your hands.

One last thing to think about, from a selfish standpoint, teaching then watching your children grow into adults using what you have taught them will be some of the best therapy you can give yourself. It's the greatest reward in life and it's at your fingertips. Don't blow it!

5

EVERYDAY SUPPORT

✦

"You Don't Look Sick"

"You don't look sick!" If every sarcoidosis patient had $1 for every time someone has said this to us or thought it about us, then we would have enough money to pay our unlimited medical bills, buy our required prescription drugs for life and still live a very comfortable life, without any debt. That phase has got to be the most repeated phase I've ever heard in regard to sarcoidosis patients. I don't know of many who have not had that said to them (except those with sarcoidosis on their skin, are in a wheelchair or on oxygen), at one time or another, whether it's by loved ones, friends, co-workers, medical professionals, Social Security personnel or we even ask ourselves. I hear it all the time along with…"I didn't know you were sick because I always see you in warm-up outfits."…"You always have a smile on your face, you can't be sick."…"You must not be too sick because I see you walking around the neighborhood."…And so on. Of course when you try and explain to them what's wrong, then comes, "Sarcoidosis? What the heck is that? I've never heard of sarcoidosis so it must not be that bad. After all, you look so healthy." Then they start looking at you with this "I don't know what to say to you" look on their face. Sometimes, no matter how hard you try, they just don't get it!

But the reality of the matter is, we are sick…Chronically sick to be exact. That doesn't mean our lives are a waste or we want you to feel sorry for us. Actually we want to be treated normally, as that's the one thing most of us miss the most…Being normal. In fact, we can still live a productive, happy, satisfying, and rewarding life. It just means that we have a chronic health condition that we must be aware of and treat on a regular basis in order to live that productive, happy, satisfying, and rewarding life. As a result of this chronic health condition, at times we need support from those "others" close to us in our life. This is yet another reality of our current life situation, so let's be honest about it.

For the most part, those "others" in our lives are our spouses. For the sake of this chapter, I'm going to refer to spouses as your husband, wife, boyfriend, girl-friend, partner, live in lover, parent, child, grandchild or whoever else is the pri-mary person in your household/life. In other words, when I refer to spouse it's the person who is by your side, for better or worse, for richer or poorer and for sickness and in health, whether you have officially taken those vows or not. This is the person who provides the primary daily support for you and probably is the most important person in your life. I know my wife is to me and to her grand-mother as well.

Support is one of the most important elements in any walk of life and can have the most impact on success or failure, pleasure or pain, happiness or sadness, life or death and every other factor you can come up with. How many times do you hear someone say when a basketball team wins a championship with a couple of superstars, "They had the perfect role players to support their skills"? Or maybe when a corporation runs an effective and profitable business the leader of the groups says, "Thank you to all of the support staff that runs the daily aspects of the business. We couldn't have done it without you." Well, when it comes to your health and well being those support factors you surround yourself with are even more important and have more of an impact than any championship or suc-cessful business. Your quality of life, or maybe even your life itself, is at stake. Aside from your Faith, which without a doubt is the most important support ele-ment in your life, your spouse is the primary player that has an effect on your daily life from a support standpoint.

For starters, you have to be comfortable with yourself because everything starts with you. Be honest with yourself and those around you, especially when you are seeking support. Not being honest can be damaging and a big waste of time for not only you, but also those trying to help you. No one understands how you feel or what you need better than you. They can imagine but never truly understand unless you tell them. Don't try to cover it up because you can only hide the truth for so long and the frustration you create for yourself by having to stretch or adjust the truth only causes you harm in the end.

Frustration is a powerful and life altering emotion! In "*ME & SARCOIDO-SIS—A LIFETIME PARTNERSHIP*" I wrote something about my wife that I now do not agree with. I wrote that the only regret I had was that she did not know me before I was affected by sarcoidosis and did not have the opportunity to know me when I was an active healthy young man, so we could have enjoyed life together while I was at my fullest. Well, after talking to many sarcoidosis patients and their caregivers I now believe that was a blessing. The number one complaint I hear from sarcoidosis patients and frustration I hear from caregivers can be best put as the patient tells it to me.

They tell me my spouse is always asking, "Why can't you do what you used to do? You don't look sick." The patient tries to answer but how can they provide an answer when most times they can't even explain it to themselves because they don't know what's going on with their bodies and minds. The only thing they can say is, "I'm trying! It's just as frustrating for me as it is for you!" The frustration builds each time something comes up that is "not like it used to be". So you see with me, since my wife met me when I was already deep into my sarcoidosis symptoms, she has nothing to compare me with…A Blessing In Disguise!

Frustration can be like a snowball rolling down a mountain that just received a fresh coat of snow…It gets bigger and bigger each time it rolls over and eventually it crashes into something causing damage. Communication is the key to stopping this avalanche! Honest communication between both parties about what you are feeling is the only way to get a true understanding of what it is the two of you are dealing with, from a relationship standpoint. This means both people talking honestly about what you feel and how this new disease "sarcoidosis" makes you feel, along with honestly listening, with respect, to what your spouse is telling you. No one is right or wrong and no judgments should be made. Just keep an open mind and do everything to understand what your spouse is feeling and do whatever you can to get how you are feeling across to them. This holds true for both the patient and spouse. Once you know what you are dealing with then you can develop a plan on how to deal with it, without causing problems in your relationship.

"Through Sickness and In Health", remember that phase? Maybe they should add, "It won't be easy" to the vow because it won't, but that is the hand you are now dealt, so you can only play it out in a positive way. Being a chronically ill patient and being a caregiver to a loved one with an incurable disease, such as sarcoidosis, is tough on both parties involved. That's why honest communication and understanding of each other's feelings is critical to the success of the relationship.

As a patient we already know it's hard, common logic tells us that. You are feeling the pain and your quality of life has changed, with at times life itself at stake. Chronic pain and fatigue can cause many problems, especially from a mental aspect when you must deal with the fact you can't function the way you once did and the uncertainty of your future. But please remember that being a caregiver can at times be even harder, from both a physical and especially a mental aspect. It's far from a cakewalk!

First of all, from a mental aspect, it's a lot easier to feel what you are experiencing than having to imagine what a loved one is experiencing and you know there is nothing you can do to make the pain go away, only be there for your loved one. This is why I say at times it is harder mentally on the caregiver than the patient. At least we know what we are dealing with!

Caregivers must be strong physically as well, because there is a tremendous amount of responsibility that comes with taking care of a loved one. There is the responsibility of carrying the load when it comes to working and being responsible for the financial end of the relationship, especially if the patient cannot work. Not only do you bring home the majority of the financials, but in addition you are probably responsible for ensuring all the bills are paid. This can be at times a heavy load with consequences at stake if you slip up. Then there is the work around the house that although we might be able to help out with in some ways now and then, these chores have to be done on a regular basis, and again the majority of the responsibility probably falls on the caregiver. One thing I do is I take responsibility for chores that I know I can do. For example, I wash my own clothes and keep the towels/wash clothes washed and put up, along with paying the bills, not bringing home the majority of the monies, but actually writing the checks and ensuring the bills are paid on time (as my wife does the same for her grandmother) and doing the majority of the grocery shopping. I also make sure dinner is either cooked or have something ready for my wife to cook when she gets home. Now this might not sound like much but just knowing I will be taking care of these chores does make a difference in our relationship, although I'm sure my wife would like me to be able to do more, and has a positive impact on my mental outlook as well.

Now in addition I try to help with other things around the house when my health allows me to. Understanding my reality comes into play again, although I still do stupid things at times. I remember shoveling the snow one March day from our driveway because I was waiting on a delivery and then almost passing out, plus my ribs were sore for about two weeks. I paid the price when I should have just waited for someone else to shovel the driveway or covered the carpet to catch the snow the delivery people would have tracked in (probably the best decision in this situation). But I gave in to my pride and just knew I could do it without hurting myself...Wrong! As I've said, understanding your reality then honestly accepting what you can and cannot do is easier written than done! No matter how long you have been dealing with your chronic health condition, you still have your fantasy moments.

Sometimes caregivers have to do things they are uncomfortable with such as noticing, then addressing when we, the patient, are slipping. I've gone through periods when I thought I was being normal, but in reality I was having a mental lapse for a few months. Once everything got back to normal I would not only notice I had not paid this or that nor could I find certain things (I'm an extremely organized person), but I would have people telling me how nice it was to see me smiling again. I didn't have a clue I wasn't being my normal self! Caregivers, especially our spouses, must notice these times and take on even more of a load to ensure the family stays on course. You might have to tell us things we might not see at the time and might even be resentful towards you. But it must be addressed and in the end we will understand.

After all, it's hard to admit you are sick and not able to do what you feel you can, or should be doing. However, whatever you do, don't feel guilty about it because you can't help how you feel. Guilt is a deep and powerful emotion that serves no positive purpose. Guilt only destroys the relationship and yourself.

Guilt is something both parties must fight and be aware of. From a patient's perspective we must not feel guilty for needing help because of our health. Not to sound like a broken record but this is another reason why understanding our reality is so important. We need what we need! On the flip side we must not make our caregivers feel guilty for needing time away from us. This is extremely important for the good of the relationship. They are only human and, as I've pointed out, carry a tremendous load of responsibility on their shoulders, which they uphold because of their love for us. We owe them that respect!

Giving our caregivers a guilt-free break from us is a perfect way to let them know how much you appreciate what they do for us and from a selfish standpoint allows them to refresh themselves, so that they can continue to support us. After all if they are worn out, as human beings will get, how can they take care of us? See, when we as patients reach our breaking point we either have to take it to another level or be hospitalized. To be blunt, those are our only choices other than death. However for a caregiver they can walk away from the situation to gather themselves, both physically and mentally, then come back to continue their role in our relationship. Giving our caregivers a guilt-free break from us is the ultimate gift we can give them. I don't know about you but I would give anything to have just one day where I woke up refreshed, didn't feel any aches and pains, didn't have to take any medications and could do whatever the hell I wanted to do…Just one day! Well, we can give this to our caregivers in the form of a vacation, even if it's just for a couple of days away from us. Sure they will probably still worry about us, but at least they are away from the daily routine. I'll stress one more time the goal is "GUILT-FREE". No side comments like, "You have a good time. I should be okay." Make arrangements to ensure you will be okay, and then let your caregiver get away from you. Don't take it personally because if they didn't love you or want to be there for you then you wouldn't have to give them a guilt-free break because they would already be gone.

The same works for the caregiver. You must not make comments, give us "that" look or show us in your body language that you are fed up with supporting us. We probably already feel guilty or less of a whole human being for needing your support to start with, along with the added burden we might feel we are to you. Just like you would probably trade places with us if you could, because you hate to see us suffer, we would just as much like our situation to go away…Not just for us, but for your sake as well! It's not a good feeling to know your loved one must take on extra loads to ensure the family's quality of life stays livable. This is a major cause of depression with patients and caregivers alike.

So please be aware of your emotions and the manner in which your body language speaks to us, along with, of course, your actual words. As I've said before, nothing positive comes from guilt or lashing out. Honest and respectful communication along with the understanding of each other's feelings is the key to a successful guilt-free patient/caregiver or spouse relationship. Remember "Through Sickness and In Health"? Please do everything you can to ensure you hold up your end of the stick. You never know when the role might be reversed.

In early 2003 my wife went through a major health crisis that resulted in her having major (four hours) surgery, which by the way was successful and she has recovered great. All of a sudden it was my responsibility to be the primary caregiver for that period of time. No matter how much I've written about caregivers, until you become one in a life-altering situation, you can only imagine. Just like unless you actually experience a life-altering disease, especially a mysterious one such as sarcoidosis, you just don't know how it affects you. After all, we are all unique.

It takes you having to experience firsthand what it's like to have to care for a loved one who has a serious illness in order to truly understand the physical and mental stress that comes with the responsibility that you are responsible for the care of that loved one. As I've said many times, it takes a lot of physical effort to make sure responsibilities and daily tasks are covered, along with the mental feelings that result from the helplessness you feel at times when you know there is nothing you can do to ease the suffering your loved one is experiencing. In fact, there will be times when you are going to have to step above your worst nightmare and do what you have to do in order to ensure your loved one is taken care of. Let me give you an example of what I mean.

About five days after my wife got out of the hospital we were going to have half of her 50 staples removed from the incision left from her surgery. As we were getting ready to go, the incision started to release pus, meaning there was some type of infection in the wound. As I was sitting in the waiting room, the doctor came and got me so they could show me what needed to take place once we got home. I should have known something was up when I entered the room and my wife had this smirk on her face.

They had taken out half the staples but the incision had a wound in the middle of it that needed to be cleaned and packed daily, so the nurse was going to show us how the procedure should be done. Now as you know, and my wife knew as well, I'm scared to death of needles or seeing something going into the skin. It's just a lifelong phobia of mine. I can't even watch a needle going in someone in a movie, it just gets the best of me, no matter how much I've tried for it not to. It's just a problem (if you want to call it that) I personally have. This fact was the reason for my wife's mischievous smirk!

I sat down as the nurse first showed me how deep the wound was by sticking one of those long Q-tips about halfway into the wound. Okay, I made it through that or at least that's what I told myself. I was still okay as the nurse showed us the first step, which was to clean the wound by spraying a fluid into the wound. I still felt okay, although I knew I didn't like this at all and was getting kind of hot inside. Then it was time to pack the wound. The nurse took out a bandage and wrapped it around another long Q-tip then stuck the Q-tip into the wound and pushed the bandage down in the wound. That was my last straw!

The next thing I knew I started feeling intense heat inside my body and tingly. For some reason I started to yawn over and over (I think my mind was trying to get oxygen), as I looked away from what the nurse was doing. "Are you okay?" I heard my wife ask, as I looked up at her with a look that said, "You set me up!" The next thing I knew the doctor had me in a wheelchair pushing me outside to cool off in the Detroit March morning 20-degree weather, until I was back to normal. Fortunately, when I returned to the room the wound had been covered and my wife said she would be able to do the procedure herself, as long as I could hold a mirror for her, which I could hide behind and not watch what she was doing.

Okay, now you can stop laughing at me because there is a serious point to me telling you this story! It was a blessing that I have a strong wife who could do the procedure herself. But what if she couldn't have? It would have been my responsibility to ensure it was done at least twice a day...By any means necessary! It was a very good chance that no matter how much I tried I would not have been able to do the procedure myself. So I would have had to find a way to get it done, whether it was to hire a home nurse, find a relative, a friend or someone to get the procedure done. As the caregiver it was my responsibility and I would have had to find a way...No other choice. This would have been one of those times when, as the caregiver, I would have had to endure a heavy physical and mental stress level to make sure my wife was taken care of. My point? Being a caregiver means you have to do what you have to do and there are going to be times when it might seem impossible to achieve, but you must find a way. Another reason why we as patients need to remember our caregivers sometimes need a break from us, without guilt. After all, they have such an impact on our lives and the last thing we need is for them to be burned out. Hey, at least my wife got a good joke out of the situation, at my expense, as she told everyone she could think of. Sometimes a good sense of humor is the perfect prescription...Like I said, "She set me up!"

Outside The Home...

Although your spouse is the primary source of your support, you're not at home all the time. There are other areas of your life in which the quote of, "You don't look sick" comes into play and has an impact on your life. Friendships first come to mind.

In my opinion, if you live your life and can honestly say you have three to five friends, then consider yourself blessed. My definition of a true friend is someone who will do whatever they can for you, a person that you can communicate with openly about anything and they probably know most of your personal traits and habits. One key to the difference between a true friend and your spouse, is with your friend they will do anything they can, with your spouse they will do what they have to do. Having a true lasting relationship with a friend is just as hard as keeping a lasting relationship with your spouse. Both relationships take effort from both parties that include honest communication, trust, respect and understanding. So basically the same logic just written about, applies to true friendships as well.

But what about all of those other people in your life that you might call friends? See I look at those people as associates and the relationships you have with them are just as important from a support standpoint. The difference between true friends and associates is that with true friends you are open about practically everything in your life, but with associates you are usually close to them by way of a specific circumstance. For example, you might know them from the gym and although you might get together after your workout, your interest and conversations are usually related to the same area.

The best example of this kind of relationship is a co-worker. Think about your co-workers for a second. I'll bet even the ones you are close to, there are certain things you wouldn't dare tell them about you simply because you work together. But, you wouldn't feel funny at all telling the same thing to a true friend. See my point?

With that point brought out, a co-worker can be one of the best support factors in your life. After all, especially if you work with them on a full-time basis, you spend as much time with them as you do waking hours with your family. You have the same interest and goals, based on your common job, and have a lot of time to get to know each other as well. One thing I believe, and a lot of people are uncomfortable with this, and rightfully so, because of job-fear, is that you need to be honest with your co-workers and employer about your health. There are going to be times when you will need help and support or can't make it into the office or shop. They need to understand, to the best of their ability, what you deal with from a health standpoint. Hey, if you're not honest with them upfront because you feel they will not understand, then what are you going to do when you need their understanding? If they can't handle it upfront then you might want to consider looking for another environment that can. If you have a chronic health condition, it's just a fact of life that the time is going to come when you need support. Understanding this fact will also help ensure the business is a success, which is the real bottom line in this relationship. Personally, I would rather know ahead of time, not when it's too late, if that support was going to be there for me, when it was needed.

Now let me address something to those healthy people out there who I've heard comment, "So and so thinks they should get special treatment just because they have a health condition. Who do they think they are?" Now if you haven't ever thought that, then I know you know someone in the work environment who has. Well, here's the deal from a business perspective. First of all, it takes more resources and money to let a loyal productive employee go and hire, then train, a new employee to get them to the level of production the loyal employee was at, not to mention it's just good ethical business practice to take care of loyal employees. So if an employee gets chronically ill, but can still produce at the same level with help from the employer, then it only makes good business sense to provide that "special" support they might need. If a "special" chair will allow the employee to sit at their computer station without causing them problems, then that "special" chair will be a lot less expensive than the firing/hiring/training process. Same goes if they can be setup to work from home and still produce the same results. Not to mention it's a legal responsibility, per the Americans with Disability Act (ADA).

Having a chronic health condition, such as sarcoidosis, doesn't mean all patients can't still live a productive life and work a productive workload. Teamwork and understanding can make a major difference in an employee/employer relationship and success. The fear of honest communication must be eliminated from the workplace. How? I wish I knew. To be honest, it's going to take a lot more than me writing about the situation to make it a reality.

Support from the workplace is extremely important to a patient's life. No one should be punished for having sarcoidosis or any other chronic health condition…Period. Trust me, when I was in the corporate world I had managers who were very supportive and a manager who didn't even ask me how my surgery went when I returned to the office. It made a major difference in not only how I performed on the job, but in my personal life as well. Regardless of how much you separate business from personal, they still interact. Support from both sides, affect the performance and relationships of both sides.

It's How We Feel, Not How We Look…

You just can't put enough emphasis on the importance of positive support from a patient's, caregiver's or business perspective. When everyone is on the same page and does what they can to support each other, everyone wins. When it comes down to it, it's all about how people feel about each other and what each individual needs that's important and the key to success. After all, we are all unique as individuals, but yet we all have the same objective, to improve the quality of life for the people we love or are associated with, and for ourselves.

The fact is, it can be hard, both physically and mentally, for both the patient and the caregiver. Dealing with the same issues on a daily basis can get to anyone. Even the best relationships will, from time to time, feel like they just can't take it anymore. I've personally been there many times, as I know my wife has as well. We have never thought of leaving the relationship, as for us that is not an option, but we have been at the edge where we have felt like it just can't get any worse than this! This is normal, so be honest about it with yourself and your loved one, with no guilt attached.

The emphasis can't be on "You don't look sick", but instead on "How do you feel?" Every day will be different, but yet the same. We, as in both the patient and caregiver, must understand this and maintain honest communications between the two of us, every day. Find a way to deal with your own frustrations, without harming the other person. Now that's a hard one! But…It must be done and you must always, as an individual, be aware, regardless of how you might feel at the time. Hurting the other person does no good whatsoever.

The level of support varies from individual to individual and from situation to situation. There is no set way to provide needed support nor is there a set way to accept or ask for support. Honesty and communicating those needs are really the only way to achieve what is needed in a support relationship. We as patients must remember, we are not the only thing in our spouses lives that requires their attention and we are not the only employee our employers have to deal with, just like we aren't the only patient our doctor has either. Sometimes I think we get caught up in our feelings to the point we think we are all that matters. When you feel like some of us feel at times, why wouldn't you? Again, I know I have. This too is normal, especially when you are frustrated with how you are feeling and just downright tired, physically and more importantly, mentally. But the fact is we're not!

Expressing how we feel can be difficult for some of us. There is a fine line between expressing your feelings and coming off as complaining all the time, which turns everyone off. My wife once told me she wanted me to tell her every time I was hurting. I did this for about half a day because the reality is, I'm always hurting somewhere. Nobody wants to hear someone complaining all the time about how much they hurt. This will not only turn that person off, but when the time comes where you really need them, they might not come running as fast as they need to…The old "crying wolf" theory might be in effect. Personally, I want my wife, or anyone else for that matter, to run like a world record track star when I need help. No hesitation! Therefore I must be aware of how I express my pain, because they need to know how I feel, for which only I can tell them, but at the same time, not have my feelings drilled into their every thought. As I said, "A fine line." But the positive thing is that it can be accomplished, as my relationship with my caregiver/spouse, along with many others I know, shows. A relationship of any kind takes hard work to maintain and a patient/caregiver relationship is no different. But like all things in life…Hard work will always achieve positive results because nothing worth having comes easy. Trust me on this one; a positive patient/caregiver relationship is more than worth working for!

Positive support and the effect it has on a patient's life is the most important aspect of living with a chronic health condition and those in our everyday lives are the main source of that positive support. So keep the lines of communication open and be honest with each other. As a patient to a caregiver, please remember…"It's not how we look, but how we feel—we need you." But most importantly, and I feel I can speak for us all when I say, "Thank you for being there!"

6

<u>ORGANIZED SUPPORT</u>

◆

A Variety Of Helping Hands

In this chapter I want to touch on formal support groups and non-profit organizations specifically set up to support sarcoidosis and all aspects of living with the disease. A question I'm commonly asked by patients and their families is, "Are there any support groups in the area in which the patient writing the e-mail lives?" Actually, there are quite a few. The problem has been making those who want and need the support know they are available and how to contact them.

My views on organized support groups have changed over the years. Just after I was first diagnosed with sarcoidosis, around 1993 or so, I wanted to find others with sarcoidosis so that I could pick their brains on how they dealt with the disease. I couldn't find any local sarcoidosis support groups, and of course, I didn't know anyone personally at that time with the disease nor was I very educated myself, I just knew how I felt. At first, I didn't care about getting information on the disease or know who else was out there dealing with it because I had been through so much in my pre-sarcoidosis life that I was just happy I had something. It wasn't until I faced my reality then got over the initial depression that I became interested in what others experienced in their battles with the disease. I wanted to talk to other patients to get an idea of how they dealt with certain specific issues and see if I was really "all alone" in regard to what I dealt with. Not necessarily for personal support, but to get ideas on how to better cope with this disease…That was my primary personal objective.

After several searches I could only find a couple of support chat groups on the Internet. Unfortunately, I was disappointed with both because they did not meet my personal objectives. Instead of talking about dealing with the disease they were more into being friends and talked about everything it seemed but sarcoidosis. That was just not what I was looking for, plus nobody in the session had any suggestions about the way sarcoidosis affected me. In fact, after the sessions I felt more alone than before. I remember just after I tried these sessions, for about a month, I found out about a local support group at a Detroit medical center. My wife was trying to get me to attend, telling me that it would be good for me to be around others with sarcoidosis, but to be honest that just sounded like what I had just experienced. So being frustrated already, I declined.

From a personal perspective, I didn't want to be friends with someone or hang out with them just because we both have sarcoidosis. A person is still an individual and just because you have the same disease doesn't automatically make you friends…Just my opinion and based strictly on my personality. Instead, I wanted to communicate about our life with sarcoidosis, the pros and cons, to see if I could find something to improve the way I dealt with the disease. Now, if in turn we start to become friends, then that would be great. We would become friends because we got along, not just because we both have sarcoidosis…There's a big difference between the two. I have many friends today who are sarcoidosis patients or know someone with sarcoidosis, but they are my friends because we like each other. So unfortunately, I quit looking for any support groups.

From that time until I started promoting "*ME & SARCOIDOSIS—A LIFE-TIME PARTNERSHIP*" I just dealt with my situation the best I knew how with the resources I had available to me. I was able to talk about my situation with certain individuals during this time who were genuinely interested. One such individual was a manager I had at EDS who took a real interest in my health, not just because it affected our business relationship, but he actually was interested. There have been a few others as well and talking with someone outside my immediate circle helped a lot.

But once I started the promotions I found several support organizations that provided what I had been looking for and more. They provided outlets where other patients openly shared their experiences and the experiences of their caregivers. There were organizations that provided resources through information and other means, directly to sarcoidosis patients. Sarcoidosis awareness and the support of patients was a priority. This is what I had been looking for years ago! Although like everything in life, nothing is perfect, at least there were options out there for patients with sarcoidosis. You just have to know where to find them!

Local Support Groups…

First, I would like to touch on the topic of local support groups. By these groups I mean organized groups of individuals who are connected by way of sarcoidosis.

In most cases, but not all, they are usually associated with a local medical center or a group of individuals that use the medical facility as a meeting place, although their meetings might be held at a local library or religious facility, wherever is convenient and the least expensive, as funding is not usually available. A sarcoidosis patient who is determined to get other sarcoidosis patients together for support usually heads them or maybe a doctor who has several sarcoidosis patients looking for support. In the group, aside from patients, are, in most cases, family members or caregivers and a doctor who specializes in sarcoidosis.

Although most support groups are rather small compared to non-profit organizations, but growing as more people are aware of their existence, they can be a vital resource for sarcoidosis patients who might not otherwise have anywhere else to turn for support. They also can be of benefit to family members who can hear what other sarcoidosis patients experience and realize that their loved ones aren't unique or alone in what they feel, therefore neither are they. Caregivers need support as much as patients, in some cases. In addition, the doctors who will meet with the groups can give medical facts on sarcoidosis, making the disease more understandable, therefore less mysterious. The more something is familiar to you then the less intimidating it is and you can deal with it in a more positive manner.

These local support groups usually will have a meeting once a month in which a structured but yet informal agenda is prepared. There will usually be information of various types given out and maybe planning other activities. The information can range from sarcoidosis related material to places to get the help you might need, such as affordable day care for your children or how to contact Social Security. But the primary purpose is for patients and caregivers to express their feelings about life with sarcoidosis, as other members in the group provide support by, most importantly, listening. You just can't describe the benefits achieved when you are able to talk about your health condition to people who you feel actually understand firsthand, even if they only listen to you and give you a hug. Nothing against our loved ones or the medical professionals in our life, but the reality is if you don't live it personally then how can you truly understand? This also goes for caregivers, as they can talk to other caregivers who experience the same unique situations and feelings they experience as well.

The group gives you face-to-face interactions with others who relate to what you live with on a daily basis, therefore allowing you to put a face to the disease, other than your own. It reinforces the fact that you really aren't alone! Then during the other times of the month members can put out newsletters or plan events for the group. One major advantage this has for members is that it gives some of the members a sense of purpose again. One of the problems of living with a chronic health condition is that you aren't able to do the things you used to do. So for some of us, this means being productive again. By being involved with a support group you can take on responsibilities that fit what you can do, without the stress and misunderstanding of an employer. It brings a sense of self-pride back to a patient, regardless of how small the task may be. You can never underestimate how much of a positive influence being productive has on an individual.

A lot of support groups also try to have a yearly outing or awareness day, where they invite speakers and others from the community to just have a day to learn about sarcoidosis and themselves. It could be a picnic, luncheon or in the form of a conference. I know of some groups that meet at a hotel and plan outings just so they can hang out together without the structure of the seriousness some meetings can entail. This day is usually something the members look forward to and in addition have put a lot of work into preparing. It helps mold them together as an extended family, as sarcoidosis and what they have learned about each other, ties a common bond between them all. The sense of belonging and not being alone, for some patients, is only experienced by way of support groups. So please never underestimate or take lightly the smallest detail because that detail probably means a lot to someone. The best rule to follow…Treat everyone as you would like to be treated. In a support group environment, everyone is the same…Period!

The main problem however, for local sarcoidosis support groups, is getting the word out. It's usually fairly easy to find the local Alcoholics Anonymous meeting, HIV meeting or cancer meeting, as there are usually specific parts of the medical facility that care for these diseases. Just try finding the sarcoidosis facility in even the best medical facility or for that matter finding something on sarcoidosis posted on one of the many bulletin boards throughout the facility…Good luck. How often do you see anything on sarcoidosis in a newsletter or other material the medical centers put out? So how do you find out if there is a local support group available in your area?

The first suggestion I have is to start with your primary doctor who is treating you for sarcoidosis. He or she should know of any support groups in the medical group/facility in which they practice or at the very least know of a resource to find out if any are available in your local area. If that draws a blank then call the information line at area medical centers and inquire if they have any sarcoidosis support groups associated with, or that meet at, their facility. It's important to note that just because a local support group meets at a specific facility, doesn't necessarily mean that facility sponsors the group. The group could be sponsored by your insurance company, although this is unlikely, but maybe in the future they will take proactive approaches to patient support as my HMO does with diabetes and heart conditions, so contact them as well.

If those options fail, then try your religious organization or local charity organizations and inquire about sarcoidosis support. If you are still unsuccessful then go to the Internet and search for "sarcoidosis support groups" in your area. There are several sarcoidosis websites that list local area support groups and contact numbers. In addition, you could contact non-profit sarcoidosis support organizations (discussed next) and inquire with them. Now if you don't have a computer or access to the Internet, you can go to your local library and they will assist you in searching online. Finding a local support group might take some effort on your part but in the end it will be worth it to you and your family.

Then if all else fails...Start one yourself. If not you then ask your doctor, insurance company, or medical facility to look into it. Now I've never started a support group myself so I'm not writing from personal experience here. You could start with a non-profit organization such as the **National Sarcoidosis Society, Inc.** based in Chicago, as they have chapters across the nation. There are other non-profit groups as well that will give you advice and assistance on starting your own local support group, either under their umbrella or on your own. Just keep in mind that starting and running a support group can be hard work and once you have started the group you will have people depending on you, so please, for everyone's sake, don't bite off more than you can chew. But if you can chew the bite, then go for it because the rewards will be well worth it for not only yourself, but for the many others you will help and meet along the way.

Local face-to-face support among sarcoidosis patients and family members is a positive way to deal with the physical and mental aspects of living with this disease. Just being able to sit in the same room with other sarcoidosis patients is something a lot of patients have never experienced. You will be amazed at the results you will get from just talking and listening to other sarcoidosis patients, as at times giving advice can be as rewarding as receiving. When done correctly local sarcoidosis support groups are a win/win situation.

Non-Profit Support Organizations...

Now let's touch on the non-profit organizations that support sarcoidosis. When I refer to non-profit organization I'm referring to those organizations that have filed non-profit status (501C) with the government as an organization that supports sarcoidosis. There are several benefits to becoming a non-profit organization such as tax breaks, both for the organization, activities, and for those people who provide personal donations. Plus, as a non-profit organization you obtain more clout, therefore allowing you to benefit from programs the government might have available, be able to get more corporate sponsorships and be able to get into medical facilities easier than a local support group.

The primary objective for "most" of these organizations is to support sarcoidosis patients and their families in any way possible, although there are a very few that their only mission is to raise money for research or other functions benefiting the organization solely. In fact, I had one organization, right after I first implemented my website, when I only informed them I was putting a link to their website on my links page as a F.Y.I., and didn't ask for anything in return, respond twice with the same e-mail telling me that they are only in the business of raising money for sarcoidosis research and for me not to expect anything in return from them, "quote—unquote"! Needless to say, the next day their link was off my website. But these situations are rare, as the majority of non-profit organizations are a positive resource for the patients.

As with local support groups, most non-profit organizations have monthly meetings as well. In fact, a lot of them not only have local support meetings in the area in which they are based, but also have chapters nationally. They will also provide assistance and guidance in setting up a support group in your area if you are interested in starting one. But again, please remember if you take on this task you will have others depending on you, so make sure you are up to the task, and more importantly, have the time and energy to take on this responsibility.

Some of the benefits of a national organization are the ability to combine resources and knowledge to make improvements in the services they provide, such as monthly meetings, newsletters, websites, physician resources, provide transportation to and from appointments for those who need it, have community fund raisers that not only raise funds for the organization but raise awareness for sarcoidosis in the community as well, along with participating in local health fairs and conducting walk-a-thons.

Another function of the national non-profit organizations is to work with government officials to get sarcoidosis legislation passed to improve the legal definition for sarcoidosis and get Sarcoidosis Awareness Days passed, both on a state and federal level. This task, as is anything in the political environment, is hard and tiring work and takes a lot of effort and resources to be successful. Everyone must get involved with letter writing campaigns to your local, state and federally elected officials to make them aware of the importance of sarcoidosis legislation. If they aren't interested then use your power of the vote to get them out of office.

With numbers comes power because the vote, when used correctly, is one of the most powerful tools in America. We must use it wisely and with the numbers of a non-profit organization behind the efforts, it shows that a lot of votes could be at stake. The truth is, sarcoidosis is not a glamorous subject or one that grabs the national spotlight, at least for now, so we must make our elected officials know that although they might not get national attention, they do have votes at stake, which in reality is the most important thing to a politician because without votes they have no job. Non-profit organizations and their members can make sarcoidosis legislation a reality, if we all work together.

There are also non-profit organizations that concentrate on providing information on sarcoidosis for others to find in one location (such as Dan's **Sarcoid Life**). These organizations are valuable to patients, caregivers and physicians alike who need to gather reliable information regarding sarcoidosis. These efforts take a lot of energy, as well as funds, but in return have a beneficial outcome for people needing information on sarcoidosis.

The non-profit sarcoidosis organization is an extremely important element in the sarcoidosis community. There are actually quite a few in existence, not only in America but in other parts of the world as well. I have mentioned a couple previously and have personally had interactions with several over the past couple of years. I've written letters for the organizations, provided insight and feedback for House Resolutions, spoken at Awareness Days, conferences and provided material for programs; to name a few ways in which I've been involved. I would like to mention them all by name but I'm afraid I would leave someone out, which would be unfair, as they range from Washington State to California to Texas to Minnesota to Illinois to Indiana to New York to New Jersey to Tennessee to Florida to England to Europe to Australia back to Michigan and many more in between.

You can find non-profit support organizations, or more specifically, ones based in your local area in several ways. First, like with local support groups, start with your primary doctor who treats you for sarcoidosis. If they do not know of any, then the Internet is probably the best place to look. You can start by going to my website, as I have several links to various non-profit support organizations. Or you can do a search on "sarcoidosis" or "sarcoidosis support groups" and go from there. Either way, if you look close enough you will be able to find a non-profit organization in your area or one that is national. If all else fails then e-mail me and I'll get you to one. You aren't alone! In fact, here are a couple more.

Sarcoidosis Network Foundation...

One such non-profit organization that I've had the privilege of working with from time to time is the **Sarcoidosis Network Foundation, Inc. (SNF),** which is based in Artesia, California (Southern California/Los Angeles area). The late Earl Jacobs, Jr. originally founded the organization in 1992 under the name of The Sarcoidosis Network and held its first meeting at the New Covenant Baptist Church in Norwalk, California. Both Earl and the first secretary of the organization have since passed away from complications due to sarcoidosis. The organization was reorganized in 1996 as SNF and is currently headed by Earl's widow, Ruth.

Earl was definitely a "can do" man who never complained about living with sarcoidosis and was deeply devoted to the well being of others, especially other sarcoidosis patients. He personally researched information on sarcoidosis, wherever he could find it, and shared what he learned with others afflicted with the disease. He always carried himself selflessly, which is something we all should recognize as a trait needed more in not only today's world but in the world of those supporting sarcoidosis because we are all in this together. He worked tirelessly to encourage and motivate patients battling sarcoidosis as he himself was battling the disease on a daily basis as well. He is truly missed by those who personally knew him! I wish I could have had that privilege.

However as a result of his dedicated wife's efforts, the organization lives on and continues to help those who deal with sarcoidosis, both from a patient and caregiver perspective. SNF provides many resources such as a quarterly newsletter, regular support meetings for patients and those "others" in their lives, who are also affected by the effects of sarcoidosis from a support standpoint. SNF provides literature on sarcoidosis (in fact, Ruth was also an immediate supporter of my first book), so patients can read all the information they can then let them determine how they want to use the information they obtain, along with providing physician referrals, which is a valuable service because as we know good doctors that are familiar with sarcoidosis are at times hard to find. SNF sponsors the "Earl Jacobs, Jr. Celebrity Walk For Sarcoidosis" (walk-a-thon) to raise awareness about the disease, along with sponsoring a F.R.A.N.D. (Friends, Relatives, Associates, Nurses, Doctors) Day. SNF has an information hot line and holds an annual "Sarcoidosis Awareness and Educational Conference" and workshop; to name a few of the positive services they provide to sarcoidosis patients.

I had the honor of speaking at SNF's eleventh annual conference in March 2003 and I left that conference with a unique respect for those involved with

SNF that made me feel that special warm feeling throughout my body and soul. The first thing that struck me was the dedication Ruth has for the fight to bring awareness to sarcoidosis and believe me it's a constant struggle! Ruth doesn't have sarcoidosis herself and she is carrying on the work of SNF in the name of her late husband as President of SNF. Now, if you have never run or been involved in running an organization the size of SNF, then you have no idea of the hard work and time it takes to do it successfully, as Ruth does today and over the past several years. A lot of spouses would have given up by now, after all it's not like she's financially benefiting or has sarcoidosis herself. Not to mention it takes a lot of her personal time. I could immediately tell by the quality and organization of the conference, including the professional manner in which I was treated, that a lot of effort went into planning this event by not only Ruth but also by others involved within SNF, it was a real team effort.

As I was flying home to Detroit after the conference I started thinking about the people I had met within SNF and that's when the uniqueness hit me. Not only did Ruth not have sarcoidosis but also many friends and volunteers do not have the disease, yet they work tirelessly to reach the goals of the organization. Even the spokesperson for the organization didn't have sarcoidosis herself. Not only did I find this extremely deep but it showed me what a strong caring human being Earl must have been to not only have his wife continue to carry on his work, but his friends as well. After all, they do not personally benefit from any findings regarding sarcoidosis, as they do not have the disease in their bodies, but yet they have more dedication than a lot of other organizations that are run by sarcoidosis patients.

Think about that for a minute…How many of your friends or family members do you honestly feel would continue your dream for you and dedicate their time and effort without financial reward for that many years with no sign of giving up, after your death? Like I said, when you think about it…That's deep! It portrays, by example, such a positive message for not only sarcoidosis organizations, but for all aspects of life! Do you feel that special warm feeling inside? SNF is a perfect example of a sarcoidosis organization that achieves real positive results for its members. We could all learn from this organization!

If you would like to contact the **Sarcoidosis Network Foundation, Inc.** you can by writing to **11428 E. Artesia Blvd…Suite 10…Artesia, CA 90701** or calling **(562) 809-8500** or visit their website at **www.sarcoid-network.org**. As always, you can also e-mail me via my website and I can give you updated information if by chance either the address or phone number has changed as I keep their website link updated on my site.

Across The Big Pond...

As we have established, sarcoidosis is a worldwide disease, therefore organized support groups are worldwide as well. Such an organization that has supported my projects and I've communicated with on several occasions is the **Sarcoidosis And Interstitial Lung Association (SILA)** based in London, United Kingdom. As of this writing, it's a one of a kind organization supporting sarcoidosis patients and trying to raise sarcoidosis awareness in England. Although the first known case of sarcoidosis was noted in the United Kingdom, there is still much mystery surrounding the disease, just like here in the United States. Patients overseas have the same issues, concerns and support needs as us. The SILA is one place patients can go for support, information and assistance.

My first exposure to the SILA came in late 2002 by way of Heather Walker, who is the SILA's secretary and a sarcoidosis patient herself. She wanted to do a book review and interview so I sent her a copy of my book. Turns out she gave me a positive review, became a positive supporter and resource along with introducing me to several other SILA members with whom I have communicated with via e-mail since that time. Although our governments operate differently, or at least to some degree, but in reality politicians are politicians anywhere in the world, there are still very similar issues in regard to sarcoidosis support, understanding and awareness that we all deal with on a daily basis. In addition, the SILA attempts to work with other sarcoidosis organizations throughout Europe to help bring awareness to sarcoidosis and assist any patients or caregivers who need support. Like all of us, Heather too has an individual story to tell.

Heather was born in 1933 in Scotland and was raised on a farm. However, her father was not a farmer but instead was a works chemist in a linoleum factory, which produced bombs and equipment for the war. At the age of 14 the family moved to Edinburgh. Heather left school to work in a government laboratory until she went on a three year working holiday in New Zealand before returning to work in London, where she settled down. Heather had always been in good health, except for the usual childhood ailments, including jaundice. But around 1987 things started to noticeably change.

She started coughing up blood on a regular basis and went to see her doctor for the problem. Her doctor told her she had nothing to worry about as her X-rays showed nothing out of the norm (sounds familiar, huh?). Based on information she later researched on the Internet, Heather found that this was a rare symptom of sarcoidosis that seems to only affect women. As the symptoms continued she spent six months being tested at a local hospital, as she continued to be increasingly fatigued, started experiencing severe itching on her skin, her joints became painful when she moved, and her eyes became sore. Finally, Heather was diagnosed with sarcoidosis. Thinking back on it now, a lot of the symptoms she experienced, although not as severe as now, were present back as far as 1972. So when did she actually develop sarcoidosis? This is a question a lot of us ask ourselves and the answer seems to always be the same…Who knows?

At the time of her diagnosis she had taken an early retirement. With the chronic fatigue and other symptoms, working was difficult. Her doctors seemed to think she could still work and basically she just didn't want to. This added to the mental frustration she was experiencing. In fact, her doctor told her to get a job because that would make her feel better. Her family and friends were generally supportive. In fact, some asked their own doctors for any information or advice they had regarding sarcoidosis. But Heather's biggest fear was not being able to get a job again after she started feeling better due to her age (54 years old at the time) and her diagnosis. Like Social Security in America, getting state benefits with sarcoidosis in England proved extremely difficult for Heather.

So, as a result, she became involved with the SILA and currently works from home supporting the SILA in a variety of ways. But working on a daily basis for a sarcoidosis support organization is not an easy task, whether it's in America, England, or anywhere else in the world. However, the need for sarcoidosis awareness and patient support is needed everywhere and England is no different.

Now in her seventies, Heather is still going strong, as is the SILA. They are doing all they can to promote sarcoidosis awareness by holding Sarcoidosis Awareness Days, contacting magazines and newspapers to print information on sarcoidosis, and putting up posters everywhere they can to let others know of the organization, maybe even reaching someone needing support that thought they had nowhere to turn. They also have their own website that is updated with information made available not only to those in England, but all over the world, along with distributing their own newsletter. They are also working with their government to pass legislation to help sarcoidosis research and support sarcoidosis patients.

One interesting story I heard while communicating with Heather also shows the similarities in people and the importance people put on issues that affect them or someone known to the public, whether it's in America or abroad. The story goes like this…A politician was diagnosed with sarcoidosis and was off work for a year. The politician contacted another sarcoidosis organization in Europe and got immediate support personally and for their organization. This is a good thing and shows what positive support can do for people, but it brought on a statement from Heather that I've heard many times over from Americans. The statement went like this, "I think if politicians were also sarcoidosis patients and/ or publicized the fact then more could be done for sarcoidosis patients in general." How true is that?

Now I wouldn't wish sarcoidosis on anyone, but the fact is if a politician had a personal interest in sarcoidosis then legislation regarding sarcoidosis would get priority. Regardless of where you are, this is a fact of the political game and something sarcoidosis awareness is missing. In addition, and again I wouldn't wish sarcoidosis on anyone, if someone "famous" or "was a household name" had the disease and was an advocate for sarcoidosis awareness, research, legislation and patient support, then again we would see an urgency to make those things happen. Look what Magic did for HIV awareness, as 90% of the people know whom I'm talking about when I just say "Magic", and for those who don't I'm referring to Earvin "Magic" Johnson, the former NBA star of the 1980s and early 1990s with the Los Angeles Lakers and current successful businessman. He suffers like everyone else but by simply allowing his public name and positive reputation to be used to promote HIV awareness and change, positive change has occurred. As of early 2004, sarcoidosis just doesn't have that "worldwide" name (although there are several public and popular people that suffer from sarcoidosis or either are spokespersons for the disease) that people relate to sarcoidosis or that well-connected politician whose mission is to help sarcoidosis patients with legislation. It's just a fact of life that if the shoe is on your foot then you walk with a different strut than you do if you were barefooted. And this isn't just an American thing, because sarcoidosis patient issues, awareness and support are just as badly needed in England, Europe, the Netherlands or anywhere else in the world where a sarcoidosis patient suffers. Seems like we really do have a lot in common after all!

I know it's a big dream to hope that one day we can have a national sarcoidosis organization and database with support groups, doctors, patients and contact information so sarcoidosis patients can get help when it's needed. Sharing information is a key requirement for success. But when you think about it maybe a national network is not such a big dream after all but really a small one. Maybe we should really be looking at a worldwide network and database. In today's world and the world of the future, our world is growing smaller and smaller. With modern travel and the power of the Internet we should be able to tap into information and resources from anywhere in the world. After all, sarcoidosis is a worldwide disease. Maybe it's time we changed our thought patterns from thinking local to national to worldwide. A united world that shares information will only make living in this world a better experience for us all!

United We Succeed, Divided We Don't Accomplish Much...

United we succeed, divided we don't accomplish much...With that in mind, there is one thing every non-profit support organization seems to have as an objective, and that is they all want to have a central location for sarcoidosis patients to be able to go to for information and support. Personally I think this is a wonderful idea that would benefit sarcoidosis patients, caregivers, physicians, employers, insurance companies, Social Security and anyone else seeking information regarding sarcoidosis. A national database with information on sarcoidosis patients (as given by the patient themselves so no privacy laws are broken), doctors that support sarcoidosis, sarcoidosis legislation, sarcoidosis support groups, research information regarding sarcoidosis, medication information such as side effects, purposes and cost, are just some of the information that should be available.

But in order to achieve this goal, along with having a national network in which all non-profit organizations link together and share information and resources, all non-profit organizations must put their own personal agendas aside and work as one. After all, we as sarcoidosis patients have a lot at stake in the outcome of research and having the ability to get reliable information about our disease, treatments, benefits and support in order to make intelligent decisions about our own health lives.

No effort is too small, especially if we can tie everyone together in some type of national and worldwide network. United we can accomplish so much, whereas divided we accomplish very little. This is so important to repeat, remember and practice. Unfortunately, sarcoidosis organizations experience, on occasion, the same politics and personal agendas that other organizations experience. This is unfortunate because as one we have so much to gain and so much at stake as sarcoidosis patients. But the fact is when funding, politics, publicity and egos are involved, people will be people and just because someone has sarcoidosis or is involved with sarcoidosis research/awareness doesn't change this hard fact of reality, although I wish it did.

I'm not going to dwell on this point because no positive result would come from it. After all, everyone has to look within themselves...Each and every day. You know if what you are doing is right or just for yourself. For now, I'll just say I wish everyone involved with sarcoidosis organizations supported everyone trying to accomplish the same objectives, instead of worrying about your own empire or whatever it is you are trying to protect. Communication, sharing of information and resources are the foundations for unity, which in turn brings success. Take a hard look in the mirror and if you fit into this personal agenda mold…BREAKOUT! We need everyone on the same page. There are a lot of different approaches and avenues to getting positive results and changes, but we must share our findings with everyone. No organization is better or less important than another…There can never be too many books from patients on the market…There can never be too much information available for patients and doctors alike…And there can never be too many helping hands reaching out to those needing help! Our families and, we as sarcoidosis patients, have too much at stake for division and politics. United we succeed, divided we don't accomplish much! Please remember that!

Sarcoidosis support groups are a great way to meet others with the disease and gather information from a patient, caregiver, and doctor's perspective. Sarcoidosis non-profit organizations are an excellent way to bring about sarcoidosis awareness, patient support and legislation improvements. For example, just think once again, of the value a national or worldwide database would bring to sarcoidosis patients and doctors alike, where information regarding all aspects of sarcoidosis, patient support and medical information was readily available. A unified organization could make this a reality.

Non-profit organizations can get into doors that the average patient can't and help to bring positive change to the quality of life a patient endures. The organized sarcoidosis support organization is a vital part of this dream and the results can be a positive step in the lives of many individuals, not only suffering from sarcoidosis, but for their families as well. We need organized sarcoidosis support groups to get involved…Together…And help make a positive difference for us all. I know it's hard work and takes a lot of dedication but in the end, it really is a win/win situation for everyone!

7

CYBERSPACE SUPPORT

◆

Online Support & The Stories Behind The Efforts

Now, in today's world, we can't leave out the Internet. For some people it's a lot easier to open up about your health problems when you are communicating in the comfort of your own home without having to even use your actual name, if you choose, but instead only a screen name. It can take out the intimidation that some people feel when they talk about themselves in person, especially when talking about something as personal as your health. It can be easier to ask those sensitive questions knowing you don't have to look at the person you are asking to see if they give you some kind of funny look and you can also take your time to make sure you get the question just right, since you have the opportunity to review what you write before clicking on *send* as opposed to having only one chance to say what you mean in person.

But, in the same tone, be careful because just as it's easy for you to remain anonymous, it's just as easy for the other party to be a fraud. Like with anything…Don't believe everything you read or are told on the Internet. There's a lot…And I do mean a lot…Of information on the Internet, but that doesn't mean it's correct. In reality, anyone can set up a website and put anything they want on that site. There are also a lot of people who prey on people who are desperate for information they want to hear. Unfortunately, sarcoidosis patients can fall into that category since there is so little concrete information about our disease, although information is improving if you look hard enough. So my point is…Like with everything in life, just use common sense and be careful. There are scam artists in every aspect of life, so treat the Internet no differently.

SarcoidBuddies & Kipy...

However, when used correctly, the Internet can be an excellent tool for sarcoidosis support among patients, from not only your area but from all over the world. Regardless of what you experience there is usually someone somewhere who has experienced the same, and just maybe, they found a way to deal with it in a more positive way than you did or vice versa. Sometimes it's more rewarding to give positive advice about your experiences to others who can benefit from what you have experienced than any other kind of therapy. When you are in a position in which you need assistance, quite often it makes you feel useful again to help others, and we all need to feel useful from time to time. After all, no one can give better advice on how to deal with sarcoidosis and the effects the disease has on your quality of life than other sarcoidosis patients. We live with the disease and all of the effects on a daily basis! I'm not talking about medical advice or how to treat your condition, but advice on how to cope with the every day struggles we as patients deal with, which is really the essence of support. One such organization that provides this positive resource, and I would like to mention specifically is an online sarcoidosis support chat group that goes by the name of **SarcoidBuddies**.

Now, in order to truly understand SarcoidBuddies and the wonders it can do as a support group, which is really what it is as opposed to your "normal" chat sessions, you must first understand the background of the founder of Sarcoid-Buddies...Kipy.

Kipy was born in 1956 and resides in South Carolina. As you have read in previous chapters, a patient's pre-sarcoidosis life is totally different than life with sarcoidosis...Kipy was no different. She was a perfect example of a workaholic! Kipy faithfully worked anywhere from 40 to 60 hours a week along with teaching Sunday School for third and fourth graders, plus sang in the church choir. Energy was bubbling out of her and being around other people was her primary joy as she enjoyed bowling, skating, going to the movies and was basically game for anything that involved clean fun with other people. She was so full of life and enjoyed every minute available to her. As she put it, "Life was good!"

Then in 1990 Kipy had her gallbladder removed along with a hysterectomy that same year. At the time she was 35 years old. After the surgeries she starting feeling tired all the time and starting experiencing shortness of breath. When at work it seemed everything moved in slow motion as her energy stopped bubbling; in fact energy for Kipy was now non-existent. In addition, her left ankle swelled up for no apparent reason as she started aching all over her body. "I felt like I had been hit by a truck", was how Kipy described the feelings she was now experiencing on a daily basis. She had assumed she was still recovering from her surgeries, but something started telling her that this wasn't the "normal" recovery process.

It got to the point that her routine became come straight home after work, have her mother help her up the stairs where she would collapse into her waiting bed. While in bed alone she would cry while her body ached from head to toe. She ran a fever, but yet her body felt chills. Nausea set in while eating was the last thing on her mind and even if she thought about it her appetite said, "NO". When asked about her mind frame during this time of her life she simply says, "I felt like I was dying inside!" Unfortunately I, like many others, understand this feeling!

But on the positive side that "dying" feeling scared her into going to her family doctor. When her family doctor heard her describe her symptoms, he downplayed it by saying it was probably "just" a bug or something (reminds me of my first seven doctors telling me it was "just" sinus problems). Fortunately, Kipy was persistent about the fact that something was wrong with her and it wasn't "just" a bug. We know our bodies better than anyone possibly can, so be relentless and advocate for your health at all times; it's your health at stake and no one else's! So, although the doctor didn't feel it was necessary, he went ahead and did blood work anyway. I wonder if the fact Kipy told him if he didn't do something that she would find another doctor had anything to do with his change of heart? As I've said before, we really do have control of our own situation because we control the bottom line...$$$—our insurance dollars and our own (co-pays)!

She got a call from her doctor a couple of days after the blood work. "I can't believe you are able to stand on your feet, much less work!" was the doctor's response. "Something is definitely wrong." The results showed her SED rate (the amount of inflammation in the body) came back at 98. Based on my recent blood work results the normal rate is 0 to 15. At first the family doctor thought it was a result of rheumatoid arthritis, which is a chronic disease also of unknown origin that is characterized by pain, stiffness, inflammation, swelling and sometimes destruction of joints. So, fortunately, he asked for help by sending her to see a Rheumatoiogist for further tests. The ball had now started to roll!

The Rheumatoiogist was very supportive and showed a lot of enthusiasm toward finding what was wrong. After a few tests he discovered an enlarged hilar mediastinal lymph node near Kipy's heart. He immediately sent her to a Thoracic Surgeon's office that same day, who after examining her scheduled a mediastinoscopy two days later. The purpose of the surgery (as was told to Kipy) was to rule out lymphoma.

When it came time for the surgery there was a problem. After Kipy had gone through pre-surgery preparation the doctor came in and informed her they would not be doing the surgery that day. When she asked why they informed her that her Prothrombin Time (PTT) and Protime (PT) levels were elevated. Prothrombin is a plasma protein produced by the liver in the presence of vitamin K and converted into thrombin in the clotting of blood, which meant in Kipy's case if the surgery was done her blood wouldn't clot resulting in the strong possibility of her bleeding to death. The doctor didn't have a clue as to why her blood wouldn't clot so he sent her to a Hematologist at another hospital to get a second opinion. Well, after seeing three separate specialists at three separate hospitals, along with extensive blood work, they all agreed that there was no scientific explanation as to why Kipy's blood would not clot. After all, she had already had a couple of surgeries in the recent past without any complications regarding her blood clotting. So it was decided to postpone the surgery for three weeks and see what happens.

In three weeks, after doing nothing different except increasing her prayers to God and asking everyone she came in contact with to also pray for her, Kipy's PTT and PT levels were still elevated slightly but not enough to cancel the surgery or cause any complications. After her successful surgery Kipy received her diagnosis in 1992 that she did not have lymphoma but instead was diagnosed with sarcoidosis!

When she went back to see her Rheumatoiogist he came in, hugged her then said, "Young lady there is no doubt in my mind that you have received a miracle. I've seen lymphoma on an X-ray like that many times and was sure that was what you had." When he told her the surgeons had told him about postponing the surgery due to her blood not clotting Kipy responded, "Well, I guess God wasn't finished healing me and He didn't want them to operate on me yet and that's why my blood wouldn't clot." He smiled and said, "You know there are many times when things like this happen and we doctors have no idea why. That's why we just wait two or three weeks and go from there. But if you ask me, I'm sure God healed you of the lymphoma!"

Although Kipy currently has sarcoidosis in her lungs, joints, connective tissue, skin, lymph nodes, peripheral nerves in both legs, along with the glands in her neck and eyes…This is the main reason she doesn't complain. God does everything for a reason and makes no mistakes. God has a plan for us all; it's just that sometimes it can be difficult to understand our plan or why we go through what we do. That's why it's called Faith and is the most powerful element in the universe! I have the utmost respect for Kipy's character and the impact her positive attitude has on others she comes in contact with. She is truly a strong woman mentally, spiritually and physically!

Now just because Kipy doesn't complain doesn't mean she couldn't…She just doesn't choose to. As a result of the location of sarcoidosis (as with most sarcoidosis patients) Kipy experiences a multitude of chronic health conditions and symptoms on a daily basis. This is one reason why it's so hard to explain to others how sarcoidosis affects a patient because each individual is different based on their location and stages of the sarcoidosis granulomas in their organs or glands.

In Kipy's case she experiences chronic fatigue on a constant basis. As she puts it, "Now I'm tired all of the time! I have no energy and sleep a lot. Many times now I'm hurting so bad I don't even feel like dressing. Although I used to be very active, now I don't do much of anything. When I do go out, I get tired very easy and come home aching so bad all I can do is go to bed." Personally, I think chronic fatigue is one of the hardest mental aspects of having sarcoidosis, as a majority of patients I've spoke with suffer from the condition. Take it from someone who knows and experiences it on a daily basis, if you let it, it will drive you to the brink of madness. It's so difficult to have your mind telling you to do something and your spirit wanting to do something, but your body isn't having it. Chronic fatigue is a difficult chronic health condition to deal with. Again, it's so important to understand what you are dealing with so you can truly understand what you can and cannot do. This is not being negative or putting yourself down but instead it allows you to avoid some of the frustrations of trying to do something you can't and by understanding what you can do and pacing yourself, you can start doing things you enjoy again. Maybe not on the level you used to, but at least on some level or maybe find other things that interest you that are more within your energy levels. Please remember this if you don't remember anything else…**YOU ARE NOT LAZY! YOU HAVE A CHRONIC HEALTH CONDITION!**

Kipy tried for five years to continue working (after all she is a workaholic by nature) despite the constant pain. Accompany this with the fact her management and co-workers didn't understand sarcoidosis nor how to continue to make Kipy a valuable and productive employee, therefore it became too much to handle both physically and mentally. How many times have we seen how your employer handles an employee with a chronic health condition makes all the difference in the world? I wish business ethics were still a priority in Corporate America today. Now, before you folks start telling me how negative I am and how I feel people should be treated special because they have a health condition, let me again say that just because you are healthy and have a job today doesn't mean you will tomorrow…Think about that. What would you do if tomorrow you lost your job out of the blue or because you became chronically ill? We're not asking for special treatment or to not be held to the same work standards. All we're asking is that sometimes an employer can make adjustments to ensure a valued and dedicated employee can still be as productive as before. A person with a disability or chronic health condition can still be your star employee. Loyalty is something that should work both ways! So after 23 years of being a dedicated employee who went beyond the call of duty (remember those regular 60 weeks?) and did everything she was asked to do, Kipy left the company and went on disability.

Along with the chronic fatigue there are other conditions Kipy must deal with. Her eyes and mouth are always dry because her salivary glands and glands in her eyes don't work anymore. As a result, it's extremely difficult for her to cry and she must use lubricant eye drops every day and night. Due to the dry mouth her gums are receding and she must use a special toothpaste and mouthwash along with constantly drinking water to replace the fact she doesn't have any saliva. Her face breaks out, making her at times look like she has the mumps when her glands are inflamed. When attempting to sleep her legs constantly jump. That, combined with the pain in her legs, makes sleeping a luxury she doesn't experience often. Quoting Kipy, "I'm never without pain!" To combat the pain or attempt to keep it at a tolerable level, she takes vicadin, muscle relaxers and antidepressants. Then when the pain is intolerable she puts her faith in God.

Learning to deal with pain both from a physical and mental aspect is something that most sarcoidosis patients must learn. Whatever works for you is what you should go with because we are all different. Listen with an open mind to what your doctor suggests and maybe even more valuable, listen to what other patients do. Then you decide what works for you. Sometimes your best resource is other patients. Although the doctors, scientists, specialist, caregivers or whoever else might be involved with sarcoidosis patients have a good understanding of what the disease does or how to maintain/support it, no one understands the effect on a patient better than another patient. You simply can't understand how it feels until you experience it personally on a daily basis. Other patients are a valuable support outlet for patients and caregivers alike. In fact, this is the premise for SarcoidBuddies.

In 1998 Kipy received a WebTV for her birthday. Since being diagnosed approximately six years prior, she had yet to talk to anyone or met anyone with sarcoidosis. Like a majority of sarcoidosis patients, she felt so alone! So as soon as she signed on to the Internet, her only objective was to find someone with sarcoidosis to communicate with who could understand firsthand what she dealt with. "There had to be others in this world with sarcoidosis!" she would constantly tell herself. She posted several messages on various message boards asking for a pen pal who had sarcoidosis. She was able to meet several people that way and also heard of a chat room for America Online (AOL) users. But unfortunately with WebTV she couldn't access AOL or any other chat sessions except for TalkCity. She entered several chat sessions for chronic diseases but in those sessions she never found anyone who had even heard of sarcoidosis, much less experienced it.

So then God gave her a direction and idea. If she was having so much trouble finding others with sarcoidosis then surely there are other patients who are doing the same. At that point her main objective became to start a chat session to bring other sarcoidosis patients and their caregivers together so that they could communicate with other people who personally understand what we go through and be there to offer love, compassion and support for each other; something that is a lot of times missing in our lives. Kipy didn't want anyone to ever feel as alone as she had felt for the past six years before she got online!

She discussed her idea with an online sarcoidosis friend she knew only as Penny. Being new online Kipy had no idea as to how to start her chat room at TalkCity for the purpose of bringing sarcoidosis patients together. Penny wasn't much for chat rooms but for Kipy she would help her set up the chat session. Since Kipy and Penny would always end their communications with "Your Sarc Bud, Kipy" when Penny set up the chat room she named it "SarcoidBuddies".

Now came the hard part…Getting the word out. First she went to all of the sarcoidosis sites she knew of that had message boards and posted a message informing people she was having a chat session on Wednesday nights at 10:00 P.M. EST and how to access the chat room. She also tried having a chat session on Saturday afternoons at 2:00 P.M. EST, but that never got off the ground, at all. So she stuck to Wednesday nights as the official meeting time for SarcoidBuddies.

Still not having any success getting people to attend, she decided to form her own web page called "Kipy's Place" where she told her story, gave information about sarcoidosis and of course informed surfers about her chat session on Wednesday nights. Finally she got a break. Brenda, The Webmaster for the World Sarcoidosis Society (WSS) website, which was one of the biggest sarcoidosis websites at the time, although it is scheduled to be shutdown in 2004, as Brenda has retired, wrote and offered to help get the word out (a perfect example of how if we stand united and help each other we can accomplish so much) by posting information about SarcoidBuddies on the WSS site. She also asked if Kipy would like to be one of the facilitators at WSS and she immediately said, "Yes." Her job was to send out welcome letters to people who signed the guest book when signing on to the WSS website. Kipy designed the letter and, of course, included information on SarcoidBuddies along with inviting everyone to join her on Wednesday nights.

In the beginning there were too many nights to count where Kipy would just sit at home alone in front of her WebTV waiting for someone, anyone, to join her as the lonely feelings increased with each passing minute until at 11:00 P.M. she would sign off and go to bed. But even though she would be down because no one showed up she kept telling herself that she was like the guy in the movie "Field Of Dreams" who kept hearing, "If you build it, they will come." With determination, a lot of prayers and unconditional Faith that this was a reason God healed her years ago…Eventually people started to come! Then TalkCity went under and she was forced to move SarcoidBuddies to another provider, Microsoft Network (MSN). Luckily Kipy had just bought a computer so SarcoidBuddies was still alive and well. Like in "Field Of Dreams", eventually people did start to come!

In April 2003 SarcoidBuddies had their official four-year anniversary with over 250 regular worldwide members and still growing each weekly session, as by yearend they were over 350. There's now a SarcoidBuddies message board where patients can post messages, questions, feelings, symptoms or anything else plus have the option of having replies sent directly to their e-mail address or simply post on the message board. There's also a calendar where members can post their birthdays, anniversaries or events of interest. It's truly a patient friendly support organization!

But what makes SarcoidBuddies so special is the unstructured but organized format of the chat session. It gives everyone an opportunity to open their minds about what you experience in your daily lives and provides support that's different from any other chat session or in-person support group, which technically is what SarcoidBuddies really is…An unstructured support group run by sarcoidosis patients, for sarcoidosis patients, and their caregivers. In other chat sessions there is usually a guest facilitator and main topic, which limits the chat discussions to a certain degree. However, with SarcoidBuddies, any subject is open and you can even go into a private chat room if you desire. Plus, as mentioned previously, an advantage of an online chat as opposed to an in person support group is you can remain anonymous if you like, which also makes for a more open line of communication. It's a lot easier for most people to sit in the comfort of your own home without facing others and ask questions you might otherwise be ashamed to ask. There are no looks of disapproval or uncomfortable body language, plus online you can take your time to carefully write what you want to say. There are members who get together during the year and there are members who are only known by their screen name. It's strictly up to the individual. Whatever works for you, so you can truly have a positive experience!

I would personally and do constantly suggest SarcoidBuddies to the many patients I come in contact with, either in person or via the many e-mails I receive. So far I've only received positive feedback from those who have took my recommendation. I once asked Kipy where would she like to see SarcoidBuddies in the future. She responded by saying, "There are other chat rooms that are mostly to inform the sarcoidosis patients of information about sarcoidosis, which is great. At SarcoidBuddies, even though I try to pass on useful information that I find, we are mainly just there to offer support, love and compassion so that no one ever has to feel alone and I would like to see it stay that way." I think that sums it up…Don't you?

You can access SarcoidBuddies by going to the links page on my website or e-mail me for updated access information. You could also do a search for Sarcoid-Buddies as well. Once you are there just click "Join" and in a few minutes you are a member. Oh, one last important note…There is no charge to join SarcoidBud-dies, no membership fee nor will anyone try to solicit funds from you or sell your e-mail address. It really is a patient support group!

Sarcoid Connection & Luiggie…

Another excellent source of information and a support outlet comes from an Internet resource that goes by the name of **Sarcoid Connection**. The site was created and maintained by a sarcoidosis patient named Jose, who is known by his friends as Luiggie. Just like with SarcoidBuddies, it's important to first understand the story behind the creation and thus giving you a better understanding of the objective for the website/support outlet and current status.

Luiggie was born in Puerto Rico in 1959. As a child he was never able to compete with the other kids, as he was always getting tired and coughing, even at a very young age. Although he was one of the fastest kids in the neighborhood, he couldn't run any distance to amount to anything without being out of breath, so of course he was always left behind. Because of this, he never played sports, although he did try baseball for a short while, with the same results. He told me, "Every time we played hide and seek, I would be the first one caught because I would always cough, so they knew exactly where I was hiding." So as a result, Luiggie was primarily a loner. You know how kids are…If you can't keep up then they don't have time for you.

His primary activities included going to the movies, sitting around the park scene and basically anything that didn't require any energy. The one positive thing that came from his inability to be active with the other kids is that he was able to stay out of trouble and avoid the temptations that surrounded him. But at the same time, Luiggie started feeling as if life was passing him by and in turn these feelings of being left out started to instill a "negative" attitude in Luiggie towards life in general. Just because he wasn't active physically didn't mean he wasn't active mentally, and like all kids needed to stay busy, as he was fully aware of his surrounding environment and the activities he was missing.

Luiggie grew up poor. In fact the place where he was born no longer exists, as it has now been replaced by cross roads. The next place wasn't much better. Luiggie recalls, "Our drinking cups were actually tin cans with the tops cut off. We had an outhouse and I remember a lot of mosquitoes." When he moved to New York City things got a little better, compared to Puerto Rico. He first lived on the south side of Brooklyn before moving to East New York in Brooklyn. Gangs were rampant and crime was everywhere at the time, but like in Puerto Rico, Luiggie couldn't keep up so in turn he was able to stay out of trouble.

Unlike most of the stories so far, Luiggie's diagnosis was not as cut and dry, if you can call them that, as in the previous cases. First of all, he had always had breathing and coughing problems and since in Puerto Rico he was never checked for sarcoidosis, who is to say he didn't have it from a very young age, as we have previously established children can and do get sarcoidosis. The first Luiggie can recall sarcoidosis being mentioned was around 1971 or 1972, when he was 11 years old. A doctor at a Manhattan medical center told his mother that he needed to get a specialist to treat his symptoms resulting from sarcoidosis. Unfortunately, nothing was ever done about it. Luiggie suspects his mother wasn't sure what to do, as sarcoidosis was just a strange term to her. Luiggie regretfully says, "That was a shame, but I understand."

At the age of 14 he decided he wanted a summer job. Luiggie went to the neighborhood clinic to get a checkup and was told, "You don't need to work, you have sarcoidosis. Apply for Social Security and the government will take care of you for the rest of your life." Luiggie thought about it for a second, but quickly decided he needed to work. Doing nothing and getting paid just wasn't his character, as it was bad enough he felt he was drying up in regard to doing something with his life, as he continued to cough constantly and was always tired. He felt he couldn't just wither away his life; after all he was only 14. So he went to another clinic that was less scrupulous and told the physician his story and the fact he really needed to work. The doctor charged Luiggie $50, under the table, and provided him with a work permit, which he needed since he was only 14 years old. For that summer Luiggie worked giving out lunches at the park for a day care center and, for the moment, felt productive.

That same summer he again fell ill. He was taken to a Brooklyn hospital where a bronchoschopy was performed. Once again, the result was sarcoidosis, only this time it was considerably worse. But like before, Luiggie's parents ignored the situation, as it was obvious they didn't understand the seriousness of sarcoidosis and Luiggie's health condition. Luiggie now says, "I don't blame my folks, but if they had taken a bit more interest in this matter then things might have been easier for me later on in life." With everything Luiggie had been through in his young life, he maintained a positive outlook towards his future, a trait I personally don't know if I could have maintained.

Once Luiggie became a working adult and still needing treatment to contain the sarcoidosis, he felt he couldn't start treatment because he couldn't afford to miss a day of work. So now he had only himself to blame for ignoring his health and life situation. About this time the positive outlook on life slipped, as he started doing things he had never done before…Stupid things we all do when we don't have a care in the world or care about the consequences. Things we are not proud of, Lord knows I have enough of those things in my past, but still they are things we each must live with and deal with in our own way. Although they might hurt us physically and from an opportunity standpoint, they also make us stronger and give us a better perspective on life, once we come back to our senses. Luiggie was no different.

In 1994 he met a wonderful woman and they were married on Christmas. They now have two children that they are very proud of. His wife has been an unconditional supporter and blessing for Luiggie. She was the reason he started his treatments, as she would literally drag him to his appointments. Once there she would openly tell the doctor whether or not he was taking his medications or not, something Luiggie should have been doing himself, as honesty with our doctors is critical to the success of our treatments. This would usually result in a lively discussion between them once they left the doctor's office. As a caregiver this is what she should have done and deep down Luiggie knew she was right.

She works as a housekeeper for residential clients. However, she leaves home late so that she can drop the kids off at school, allowing Luiggie to not have to get up early and go out in the cold. In addition, she does the shopping, including bringing everything upstairs to put up. Luiggie will ride with her at times, but usually just sits in the car and waits. She will call home from work about 10 times a day to check on him and make sure everything is okay or to see if he needs her to come home early. Although he has friends and family whom he can count on, if he calls them, she is the only one who is always there for him and goes out of her way to make sure she is aware of what he might need. Luiggie had this to say about her, "Although we might argue, rant and rave, she is always there. I'm one of the lucky ones to have someone like her in my life, nagging or not (he says with a smile). She gives me hope and the strength to go on with life. I owe what little bit of sanity I have left to her. If I could put into words what she means to me it would simply be put as, "I love you hon, thanks"."

His kids also are aware of Luiggie's health condition and keep an eye on him. Both kids know how to dial 911, something we as adults, with or without a chronic health condition, should make sure our children know how to do. Another thing his kids know how to do is bring him his oxygen tank when they see him coughing more than normal. Like I wrote earlier, it's important to make sure our children have the best understanding possible of our situation. You never know, they might be the only ones who can save your life.

Since Luiggie has became sicker and the sarcoidosis has become more aggressive, he finds himself more depressed than normal. The mental aspect can really get to you in ways others might not consider. For example, although he likes to be with his wife and get out sometimes, he finds it difficult to go shopping with her. Having to watch her carry all of the packages while others stare at him and obviously wondering in their minds why his lazy butt isn't helping his wife can be hard to take as a man. But the truth is, he gets winded just going to the restroom at home, not to mention that oxygen tank is not the lightest thing to carry around with you at all times, so the reality is he is doing good just to be out. But unfortunately people think without thinking at times, as some situations are not what they seem when you are looking in from the outside. In fact, my wife can give another example of this unfortunate trait we humans have. Just after my wife had major surgery and was out for one of the first times at a department store, she was slowly walking to her car, as she was still recovering and just happy to finally be outside. A car was trying to rush her up to get to her car so they could get her parking space, so they kept blowing their horn for her to hurry up, not realizing her situation, even though she would just look at them and throw up her hands. Again, thinking without thinking! However we aren't going to change human nature anytime soon so for now all Luiggie can do is try and ignore the stares.

The only thing that really matters anyway is what his wife thinks, but of course that is easier said than done.

In 1995 Luiggie was put on the lung transplant list for a bilateral transplant. At that time he felt he had less than two years to live. However, the hospital staff decided that he was too ill, therefore too weak, to survive a lung transplant, so he was placed on the inactive list. The many tests made him feel like a guinea pig and didn't make him feel any better health wise either. He was told in order to get back on the transplant list, he needed to get a little stronger in order to have a better chance of surviving the operation. To his own surprise he did indeed get stronger. In fact he got so much better that it was declared he didn't need the transplant, so here he was in limbo again…Not well enough to improve his ability to breathe and to strong to have something done that would improve his ability to breathe more normally. Then it was decided that a lung transplant was out of the question anyway, because of the fear sarcoidosis would just attack the new lungs. The Catch 22 ended with no hope!

Pneumonia has also been a problem for Luiggie. There was a time when he would be admitted to the hospital every six months or so with a case of pneumonia. Fortunately, as of late, the pneumonia has not been a major problem. Luiggie credits this to him taking it easy and accepting his reality with more honesty.

There are days when Luiggie can drive his own car and move around like nothing's wrong. Then there are those days when getting around is a dream. Even getting a breath of fresh air becomes a luxury, especially in the inner city where on some days fresh air is alien to us all. He has available to him a scooter, cane and walker to assist in getting around. A home attendant provides help around the house and is someone Luiggie really appreciates.

From a medication standpoint, he receives gomoglobulin infusions every three weeks, takes prednisone and xanax for his panic attacks, which can, to Luiggie, be worse than the sarcoidosis itself. Sometimes it seems that the treatments and side effects have a more negative effect on us, both physically and mentally…But what can we do? Without the medications, the sarcoidosis will take us down. This is just another reason for the importance of research into new, more effective ways to treat sarcoidosis and why it's so critical. The quality of life for a lot of people is at stake, not to mention for some, life itself.

At this point in his life, Luiggie honestly says, "I'm feeling like these will be my last days here. I'm not saying this for pity; I'm just being honest about what I feel and to myself. This is very frustrating, because you don't know what to do. I'm trying to get all my things in order, but my condition is not letting me. How do you tell your loved ones that you're getting ready for this?" Although Luiggie looks at his situation from a reality standpoint and tries to prepare himself for all possible situations, he continues to live life the best way he can. It's because of this attitude that Sarcoid Connection was born.

As Luiggie was getting more and more depressed, with little hope of getting better and in his mind preparing to die, he decided he wanted to help others understand what sarcoidosis was or at least see if there was a place for sarcoidosis on the Internet. After all, although writing and doing work on the Internet can be tiring, it didn't take a lot of physical involvement, so for Luiggie it was a perfect outlet. He joined a site for lung transplant patients and started chatting with the hostess. Since this site was more geared toward pre and post transplant patients, Luiggie decided to start his own website for sarcoidosis patients.

The more he researched the more he found he needed to learn about his disease, as there was more to sarcoidosis than just pulmonary related problems. The only medications he was aware of were his own, not realizing there are many others used to treat symptoms for sarcoidosis. There was so much information that needed to be made available to sarcoidosis patients and Luiggie took it upon himself to make this information available to as many people as he could in any way he could.

He already had some contacts by way of the support group he attended at a Manhattan medical center, the one he uses for his treatments. After establishing his website and online support group, it was time to get the word out. He first contacted several large corporations to see if they wanted to donate promotional items, no matter how small, to help promote sarcoidosis awareness and distribute to his members…None did. He added links to other sites relating to sarcoidosis, lung disease, Social Security, medical supplies and anything else he could find that might apply to a sarcoidosis patient.

On his own, he used his computer skills and desire to make t-shirt transfers and calendars, both with the sarcoidosis logo, then sent them to members. He made personal calls, if he had their phone number, to patients when they were ill or having a hard time. If he had their address, he would send Christmas cards, informational flyers, not only to sarcoidosis patients but to their family members as well, toys for their kids if they could not afford them (although this was not a luxury for Luiggie to purchase them either), or anything else he could think of at the time. He spent time going to stores around Christmas asking for toys or t-shirts to send to sarcoidosis patients, while explaining to the store owners about his support group and sarcoidosis…But like the major corporations, none cared to participate. Luiggie explained why he took this approach by saying, "You may think these things will not help sarcoidosis, but it's showing them they're not alone and based on the responses I've received, I can assure you a little detail like that goes a long way."

He has had members send him checks to help in his efforts, that he in turn puts towards shipping costs, ink for his printer and for the other things he sends out. He receives get well cards from members when he was having hard times, that by the way made a big difference in his mental outlook at that time. As time goes on his chat sessions are getting bigger and more informative as the Internet, if used correctly as Luiggie is doing, touches a lot of people who might not otherwise have access to this kind of information and support. Bottom line…Patients supporting patients at its best!

His future goal is to make Sarcoid Connection a real non-profit organization with sarcoidosis informational materials available to send out to anyone who requests them. He has sarcoidosis awareness t-shirts, ribbons and caps for anyone who would like to wear them, along with possibly cups and daily planners with sarcoidosis awareness and information on them. He would also like to have books and other published materials readily available, all at a reduced price since a lot of patients can't afford to purchase these materials because of the expensive medications and no health care insurance that they personally endure. All of this information and merchandise to support sarcoidosis awareness would be available at anytime, by way of the Internet or direct mailing. As Luiggie says, "I want them all wearing sarcoidosis awareness t-shirts and ribbons so that people will ask, "What is sarcoidosis?" They do ask and with the right information, you can answer as well."

Another idea he came up with recently, to give members something productive to do with their time and raise awareness, was the creation of the "Sarcoidosis Awareness Traveling Quilt". The quilt is a mission of love for Luiggie and he takes extreme personal pride in its creation. He tells me, "It's designed to show that sarcoidosis comes from all over the world, from all kinds of life, without boundaries. That's why we ask that the state or country be placed on the square."

The hope is to use the quilt to help raise, not only awareness for sarcoidosis, but to also help raise funds for Sarcoid Connection so Luiggie can continue to provide the materials mentioned at no charge or for a donation to sarcoidosis patients and their families. The quilt would be used for display purposes only and could travel around to specific events, sarcoidosis related and others as well. Anywhere that it could be displayed to draw awareness for sarcoidosis. In fact, another quilt is already being designed for those patients who have lost their lives as a result of sarcoidosis. Luiggie proudly proclaims, "My hope is one day this quilt will be famous, as others for other causes have, and will make a positive difference in peoples lives. This is why I treat it as my baby!"

Although sarcoidosis has been part of Luiggie's life for as long as he can remember, he maintains a positive and helping attitude. Sarcoid Connection is his way of getting sarcoidosis information to patients, families and medical personnel, as we all need as much information as we can get. But most of all it's a way of sarcoidosis patients helping other sarcoidosis patients and their families. The impact is greater than you might think.

In 2003, Luiggie drove 15 hours non-stop to attend a sarcoidosis conference in Indiana. There were also 14 others who are members of Sarcoid Connection, who attended as well. Not only did they want to attend the conference, but most of all they all wanted to meet each other in person. This was a beautiful experience for Luiggie personally, as he got a firsthand view of the positive impact he had made with all of his hard work. This is something I can relate to because it's a lonely feeling to be by yourself working away on your computer with no feedback or real idea if you are having an impact or not. At times you wonder if you are making a difference or just wasting your time and effort. Then when you have someone thank you and tell you that you have helped them in their life…Well, that's why we do what we do! Keep up the good work, Luiggie. You do make a positive difference!

I completed this story and had it approved by Luiggie in January 2004. He was excited about the possibility his story would be in print soon and he could sit down and read about himself in a published book, hopefully having a positive impact on other sarcoidosis patients and their families as well. Unfortunately, that will never happen. On March 13, 2004, Luiggie passed away due to complications with sarcoidosis.

Luiggie struggled with this disease practically all of his life, but yet he touched so many people in such a positive way. This was a sure sign of his inner strength and he will be missed by a lot of people, especially his loving family. This is evident by the many touching messages displayed on Internet message boards in regard to his death. As I've said before, when someone so close to you passes away from sarcoidosis, it really hits home, and Luiggie's death is no different. I'm honored that I had the opportunity to meet and communicate with Luiggie on a personal level. I pray that by writing his story and leaving it as he approved it, his memory can live on forever.

I don't know where his website or support group will go from here. I will keep the Sarcoid Connection sign on to his website (**www.sarcoidosis.us**) available from the link page of my website under the title "Luiggie's New York City Site", as long as it's available. There are several other patient stories, written by the patients themselves, on the website, as there are on various websites as well. The more actual patient stories that are out there for the world to read, only makes a positive difference in the way people view sarcoidosis patients. Thank you to all of those patients with the courage to tell your story…Especially Luiggie. **Rest In Peace!**

(** Luiggie was a member of the local support group that meets at the Mount Sinai Medical Center in Manhattan. To date I do not know the status of his projects such as the Sarcoidosis Awareness Traveling Quilt.**)

Other Positive Means…

Another positive aspect of the Internet are the many message boards that are available on various sarcoidosis and medical sites. For those not familiar with message boards, they are usually in a format where you can post a question, message or give out information (although most restrict the selling of products) for others to view and respond to. The message boards are another useful way of communicating with other sarcoidosis patients anywhere in the world and get valuable information from other patients. As you know, I strongly feel patients are the greatest and most helpful source of information for other patients in regard to coping with the daily aspects of living with sarcoidosis. Sometimes you just have to live it to understand it! In addition, you can also get advice or opinions from medical professionals that frequent/sponsor certain message boards. But, again, be careful with that information and always consult your own medical professional before trying anything new…Please! If I had a dollar for all the scams I've been offered, especially after a story is aired on television, I would be a millionaire!

Compared to just a few years ago there is now a lot of information available on the Internet regarding sarcoidosis, although again, please be careful about what you believe and always consult your medical professional before trying something you heard about on the web (I can't stress this enough). There was a time in the not so distant past when you would do a search on the keyword "sarcoidosis" and only a few listings would come up. Now, when you do the same search on the same search engine, you get thousands of matches (basically the search engine searches the web for sites matching the word "sarcoidosis").

Search engines are a good way to find sarcoidosis related sites. Your Internet provider usually provides one along with such current (2004) sites as Google.com or Yahoo.com. Once you find a site, most will have additional links to other related sites as well. For example, if you go to my website you can obtain links to other sarcoidosis and health related sites by clicking on my links page then clicking the site you want to visit. I wish everyone would support each other to make locating a sarcoidosis website easier for all patients or those interested in learning more about our disease. But...Maybe someday we all will learn the value of supporting each other!

In addition, a lot of the major medical centers and university medical centers now have a page dedicated to sarcoidosis, although you might have to look under the autoimmune disease section or go through several links to find it. Some are actually very good and then some are rather useless. I guess it depends on how much the medical center is involved with sarcoidosis or if any of the physicians associated with the medical center are involved in sarcoidosis research and/or treatment. But compared to just a few years ago, the information is improving.

The Internet is a powerful worldwide tool that will only become more powerful in the future. So if you are not familiar with the Internet, you might want to start getting used to it because it's the wave of communication for the future. In today's environment the cost is not that great and learning the technology is not that difficult as the makers of personal computers and Internet providers are making the technology user friendly so everyone can benefit from the Internet. If you can't afford a home computer then visit your local public library as they usually have computers that access the Internet available for use along with someone who can assist you. The Internet is not just for computer geeks anymore; in fact there isn't anything the average person can't research on the web. So don't be left out, there truly is a world of information and support waiting and available for you at your fingertips!

8

$\underline{21^{st}CENTURY\ INSURANCE}$

◆

It's Your Money & Health At Stake

Insurance, whether it's private, through your employer, or via our government can be a detailed and complicated process. I've seen a lot of different scenarios over the years while supporting a national health care claims system that provided national corporations such as the Big Three Autos, Kmart and others with coverage for their employees. I supported the system in a data center, financial and business analyst environment. More importantly, I'm a patient who is required to use my insurance policy on a regular basis, ranging from prescriptions to doctor visits to referrals to getting diabetic testing supplies to emergencies and so on, as anything medical requires insurance. As a result I understand both the business and personal side of how the health care claim process "really" works. So again, I'm not going to quote you a lot of statistics or refer to publications that tell you what they feel you should do to make the process easier but instead just give you my experiences and opinions for you to decide for yourself. Hopefully you can benefit from my situations.

First, I want to stress the most important thing you need to do in regard to your insurance coverage…**MAKE SURE YOU UNDERSTAND YOUR POLICY!** This may sound simple and obvious but believe me it's not. I can't count the number of times I've heard patients in doctor offices or received calls as a Business Analyst from patients who do not have a clue as to what is covered and most times this comes after the fact, as they are looking at large out of pocket expenses for procedures that aren't covered in their policy. As you know, every doctor's office and medical facility has a big sign that reads, "It is the patient's responsibility to understand your insurance policy and the patient is responsible for any fees not covered by their insurance policy." Not only is the sign posted in full view but you also sign a form the first time you see a doctor or have services at a medical facility that states the exact same thing…The patient is responsible for all fees the insurance company does not pay…You, the patient, are legally liable. So you must understand beforehand what is covered by your specific insurance policy at the time you are getting treatment. Not the year before because covered benefits change each year, in fact they can change mid-enrollment period. So you, the patient, must stay on top of your policy!

The policy is written complicated and there are a lot of little specifications that vary from policy to policy and from area to area. After all, in reality, it's a legal document and every single word and line can have an impact on your coverage and more importantly your out of pocket expenses. Make it a priority to get all of the information you can beforehand and read it. Please take the time before you enroll because on most jobs you are stuck for the year once you enroll, so again please take the time beforehand! I can't stress this enough!

Also don't go it alone. Make sure your spouse or caregiver is involved in this process because you never know which one of you will need medical attention and the other one needs to understand your benefits or at least know where to get the correct information. Even your dependants should at the least know where to find the insurance policy information and know where to find a number to call, if needed. Preparation by all parties is of extreme importance because in emergency situations there just isn't the time or the frame of mind. Plus it's just a fact of life that even if you are perfectly healthy today, the next minute you could be in a life altering situation and your health needs changed forever. Be prepared!

Then sit down and honestly determine what is the best coverage for you and your family's health care needs, keeping in mind the possibility of the unexpected. Try to minimize your coverage for what you feel you need because like anything else you are paying for all of the extras that you might not need during the upcoming year. Are you in need of specific medications, are you expecting a child, do you feel some type of surgery might be coming up, do you have enough money saved to cover a higher co-pay or emergency, if needed? Questions such as these are what you need to be asking yourself beforehand, not after you are facing high doctor or pharmacy bills.

Now in a fantasy world, wouldn't it be great, or better put…Fair, if you could get a refund or at least a percentage back if you don't use a benefit; similar to roll-over minutes that you pay for but don't use on your cellular phone bill? At least cellular phone companies are seeing the light. But we're not talking fair, we're talking insurance and although you don't get back what you don't use it's mandatory you have insurance coverage to obtain service in health care whether medical or dental, legally drive an automobile or even get a mortgage on a home; you have to obtain insurance coverage. That's just how it is in America…Insurance is the biggest legal racketeer there is! So try not to overdo it because unfortunately if you don't use it you don't get anything back.

In addition, do not forget or downplay the dental coverage portion of the policy, which although is usually included in your options/benefit dollars, is usually covered by a different insurance company. Again honestly look at what you feel you and your family might require. Do you have children needing braces or are you having problems that might need some work such as root canals or oral surgery? These are the type of questions you need to ask upfront.

What you might want to do is ask some of your co-workers if they have been satisfied with a particular insurance company, but make sure they actually used some of the benefits. That might sound too simplistic but they might have only used the policy once for an office visit whereas you are looking at the possibility of surgery or chronic care…A big difference. When I was in my pre-sarcoidosis diagnosis stage and very frustrated with the lack of positive results I was getting from the previous six doctors, my manager highly recommended a doctor he used. The experience with that doctor turned out to be a nightmare and come to find out my manager (who so highly recommended this doctor) had only seen him once for a physical. I've never forgotten to ask the important question again…"How did you use the doctor or policy?", when asking others for a referral based on their experiences.

Referrals and the referral process are big deals as well, especially with Health Maintenance Organizations (HMOs). For me my main physician is my Endocrinologist so I determine my other doctors, including my Primary Care Physician based on the same network as my Endocrinologist works out of. Your Primary Care Physician (some HMOs call them Personal Care Physicians or just PCPs) must refer you to any specialist, therefore make sure the specialist you need such as your Pulmonologist, Dermatologist, Endocrinologist, etc. is in your Primary Care Physicians network or else you can't see them unless you pay all of the fees out of pocket, although some plans such as a Preferred Provider Organization (PPO) allows you to visit any specialist without a referral, however you will pay a higher fee upfront. This is extremely important if you want to see a specific doctor. You'll hear in the advertising how you can choose from hundreds of doctors…The doctor of your choice. Well, it doesn't matter how many doctors you can choose from if the one you want and has taken care of you for years is not one of the choices. Not to sound like a broken record but…Make sure beforehand!

Then once you have made your decision and enrolled, stay on top of your policy because as unfair as this may sound, your benefits and cost can change (legally) throughout your policy even though you can't get out of the policy you choose until the next enrollment period, usually the following year, even if the policies do change and affects you negatively. Never assume something is covered, even if you have had the same procedure or gotten the same medication during this policy period, it could be different or not covered any longer. Question everything you don't feel 100% is correct, regardless of how small it is. Do not depend on others such as the doctor's office, Pharmacist, lab technician, administrator or anyone else to just tell you something is not covered or the cost they give you is correct. It is your responsibility to ensure you receive the correct benefits from your policy and yours alone! After all, you are ultimately the one who is responsible for payment.

It's not that those professionals are trying to get one over on you, trying to get out of doing additional paperwork, don't want to be on hold while making follow-up calls for you or maybe they just don't care, although to be honest sometimes those examples are the case, but not usually. Most of the time it's an honest mistake. After all, they do have a lot of patients and a ton of paperwork but then again that is the job of their choice so that's not really an excuse, just reality. The most common mistakes are just lack of communication and simply entering the wrong procedure code or submitting the wrong claim form. Then it sits on someone's desk for various reasons until you (the patient) are sent an incorrect bill and it's up to you to wade through the mess. After all, you are responsible in the eyes of the law to pay the bill. Remember that sign posted in every doctor's office, clinic and medical facility you go to? So question everything!

And please do not blame the doctor because nine out of ten times they don't have a clue as to what is being billed or not. They have enough to think about dealing with patients. However, if you do have problems with the staff, make sure you copy the doctor on correspondence so they can be aware of their staff's actions. Most hospital or medical center staff is provided by the facility, so the doctor has no control over who is hired but can take action if problems exist, whereas those physicians in private offices do control their staff hiring. So don't leave or blame a good doctor based on their staff's actions without first making them aware. Your health is too important to miss out on a physician that is treating your health in a positive manner and you are comfortable with them just because of issues with their staff, who probably won't be there much longer anyway. Now if no positive changes occur, or you feel your doctor is strictly a HMO doctor (a term I use for those doctors who are primarily concerned with seeing a specific number of patients so that they can obtain a bonus at year-end from the HMO for following the "rules", as opposed to their primary concern being to ensure their patients are treated with the proper care regardless of how long it might take), then you might want to consider making the switch. My point is…Just make sure the doctor is aware of any hassles you receive from their staff because if you don't let them know then how can they make it better for their patients? In today's medical environment the doctor is just one of many individuals involved with your health care and cost. Honest and open communication between the patient and doctor goes beyond just your physical health and mental state of mind. Today's medical processes are more complicated than that! So stay on top of your entire situation because again…It's **your** health and money at stake!

Advocate For Yourself…

Now I know this is going to be frustrating to read and even more frustrating to do but…Even after you have done everything the right way it is at times still going to be on you to make sure you get the correct benefits in which you are entitled. This will mean you might have to make phone calls to your insurance company (and probably be on hold for quite a while after several prompts) then make additional follow-up calls, maybe file an appeal regarding a benefit with your doctor's notes, get the correct procedure code from the insurance company to provide to your doctor's staff and you will probably do these things multiple times. Don't give up or get too frustrated because it's your money and rights that are at stake here, no one else's. There are going to be times that you must advocate for yourself and your family. It might not technically be your responsibility but in reality it is! It's your policy, money and health we are talking about here, remember that at all times. That fact can't be repeated too many times.

Although I could give you a whole book of examples where I've had to advocate for myself over the years, I'm only going to give you four separate situations. Now in my case I have four advantages. The first is I make sure I understand my policy beforehand so when I start researching and following-up I have a good idea of what I should be receiving.

Second, since I worked in the claims field for over 14 years I also understand what goes on behind the scenes and most times what needs to be done to correct my problem, I just need someone else to do it since I do not manage their actual system. I make sure when I start my conversation that I mention this fact before the runaround starts and each time I can tell a difference in the way the person on the other end of the phone, whether it's someone from the insurance company or doctor's office, starts talking to me. Definitely with more respect! Being able to talk intelligently, respectfully and calmly during conversations dealing with problems will not only save you time, but will speed up your results. You don't need experience in the insurance industry to get this respect, just know your policy and deal with the person on the other end of the phone or on the other side of the desk with respect. After all, we are all human beings and common courtesy goes a long way.

My third advantage is that my wife works in Human Recourses at a major Detroit Medical Center so she also has an inside understanding of benefits and can give me advice on issues I don't understand or that have changed since at this time we are on her coverage. But you too can have the same understanding by again just comprehending your policy to the fullest. This is so important!

Last but not least…I'm a very patient man! I will wait on hold or call back and will not take no for an answer when I know I'm right. It's a matter of principle with me, as well as I don't have money to double pay my insurance company and the medical professional. The ability to be patient is a very important trait to develop in life. After all, when you have a chronic health condition, waiting and follow-up is now a part of your life. Accept that fact then don't let it stop you from getting what is rightfully yours…Period!

My first example used to happen a lot and although it's really simple with a simple solution, I've spent more time than you can imagine and a lot of times ended up at a collection agency because of it. However, each time I've come out of the situation not paying a penny, which was the correct conclusion. Every other week I get an injection of depo-testosterone. The process is I bring my own medication and the nurse at my Primary Care Physician administers the injection (gives me the shot). Based on my insurance policy this is a covered benefit with no co-pay and should be submitted with the procedure code that states "injection administration". However, on more than one occasion, the doctor's office will submit the procedure code for "office visit", which costs me (unjustly) a $15 co-pay and gives the doctor an office visit charge to the HMO. This would happen even when I would provide them with the correct codes beforehand, since I had experienced this problem in the past. I would have to continue to call the insurance company, who would in turn fax a request to the doctor's office, who would in turn send in the correct procedure code. Sometimes this would take several attempts (I don't know why) and even get to a collections agency where I would again have to explain the situation, usually with a letter, which I saved online and used each time, since each time it was the same situation, just a different date. Eventually the charge would be taken off but it took up a lot of my time and effort on my part.

Currently, I do not have to worry about this anymore (although it did happen once when a new office assistant was hired) because my Endocrinologist offered to have his staff give me my injection and not bill me since my insurance policy requires my Primary Care Physician give me the injection. These are the little things that make a medical professional exceptional. The consideration for his patients instead of the $6 or so (approximately $156 annually) he would get from the insurance company for administering the injection every other week. So, thank God I haven't had to deal with this situation in a while!

My next example is in regard to emergency room visits. Now anyone who has ever had to use the emergency room (unless for maybe a serious automobile accident or heart attack) knows it can be a long and frustrating experience, especially in the inner city. There are times you will wait for hours on end, especially if your situation is not considered "life threatening". Now I understand the emergency room environment is a very stressful and critical environment where life and death decisions are made on the spot. It takes a very trained and unique individual to succeed in this type of environment and I have the utmost respect for the professionals who save peoples lives on a daily basis. But…That doesn't mean there are not serious problems with the process and how patients are treated, especially those who have to use the emergency room because of lack of proper insurance coverage. In my case not having my medical history can be a life threatening or at the least a life altering experience. This is why I can't stress enough to not only keep a detailed card with your medical information and medications on you at all times, along with using a service such as MedicAlert, but also just as important make sure your caregivers, co-workers or anyone else you are around on a regular basis is aware you have this information on you, because in an emergency situation you might not be able to communicate for yourself. Please don't be ashamed to tell those close to your situation because if you are not prepared it could cost you your life!

Now on this night this situation actually involved my stepdaughter. At the time she was in her mid-teens and was experiencing fever and an extreme sore throat. It was around 8:00 P.M. or 9:00 P.M. and my wife decided to take her to the emergency room, especially since her throat was starting to swell. One thing about my wife is that she would not hesitate to take our daughter to the emergency room. She would say in a second, "We're going to emergency!" Today we both joke with her about this all the time as we will look at her and ask, "You need to go to emergency?" But the reality was that she was a great mother and you can never be too careful when it comes to children or teenagers and their health…Better safe than sorry, as the saying goes.

On this occasion when we arrived at the emergency room, as usual it was crowded as most inner city emergency rooms are. After we waited for several hours then a while longer once we were called back, the doctor came in. Within no more than three minutes at the most he had determined she just had a sore throat and told her to take a couple of Motrin and she would be fine then he was off. The next day after no improvement we took her to her primary doctor who took one look and saw she had a serious throat infection. She prescribed some medication and couldn't believe the emergency room doctor could not see the infection since it had obviously been present for a while and without a doubt the night before. She was furious and I better not repeat the things she went on and on about.

The bottom line is I went home and called my insurance company. I explained the situation in detail and told them I wanted to protest the service and our automatic $50 co-pay for using the emergency room. To this day I never received a bill for the $50 nor did I ever receive an Explanation Of Benefits statement showing where the insurance company paid anything for the visit. If you feel you are mistreated or not given the proper care, please report it in a professional manner and with as much detail as possible. Do not take it and just keep quiet because if you do not speak out then others are going to experience the same frustrations you experienced and in their case it could cost them their life. Look at the statistics, there's a lot of unnecessary deaths caused by misdiagnosis or neglect. In the real world the most effective way to make an impact and change is by hitting the checkbook. That's the power you as a patient/consumer hold. Speak up!

Now this next example is in regard to an oral surgery I had to remove a tooth that had been causing me problems for a long time and there was nothing else we could do to save it. Take care of your teeth because your dental health affects your entire body. While I was dealing with this tooth problem I also experienced other health problems that my Endocrinologist related back to the infection/bacteria this tooth was passing throughout my body. This is especially important for us with diabetes or overactive immune systems (as most sarcoidosis patients experience) because the infection/bacteria will find your weakest point and attack. I'm telling you, your dental health is of extreme importance. Don't take it lightly!

When I went for my initial consultation I was impressed by the respect and knowledge the surgeon had for not only sarcoidosis but also for the various secondary conditions and medications I was under. He agreed we needed to extract the tooth (my left bottom back tooth or #18) and with everything I had going on health wise he would need to sedate me as well. In addition, anytime I must be put under sedation my Endocrinologist requires I be given 100MGs of hydrocortisone while the procedure is being performed. The surgeon agreed with this requirement and wanted me to contact my Endocrinologist to get any additional instructions. As always, my prednisone was increased the day of the surgery then slowly decreased over the course of the next few weeks until I was back to my normal dosage. The surgeon also prescribed me with medications to take starting a couple of days before the surgery. I was pleased with the process so far, but then came his billing department.

As the office assistant was setting up my appointment it was going to be several weeks before she could get me in. Since I was in constant pain I had her page the surgeon who told her to book me within a week at his other office (he shared his time between two offices) because I needed this tooth extracted as soon as possible because of other health issues. She didn't seem too happy about adjusting her scheduling but did anyway and was able to get me in the Monday after next (it was currently Thursday). Then as she was writing up the costs and gave me my estimate it turned out to be about $365. This immediately raised a red flag because since I knew I was going to need work (in fact this was the primary reason I waited so long) we had purchased the top of the line dental coverage through my wife's employer that covered everything at either 100% or 80% at the least. Another example of being prepared and understanding what you need done health wise in advance of determining your insurance policy, when possible.

When I questioned the cost I was told that the extraction was covered at 80%, however due to the long standing policy of the dental insurance company, if you are not getting a minimum of two teeth surgically extracted then the IV sedation is not covered and I would be responsible for 100% of the cost ($250). In addition the hydrocortisone was also not covered and again I would be responsible for 100% of the cost ($75). I told her this did not seem right and could she verify this. She gave me a sour look (maybe because it was 5:00 P.M. on a Thursday afternoon) then picked up the phone and must have called a fellow office associate because all she said on the phone was, "When less than two teeth are extracted then the IV sedation is not covered, right? I thought so." Then she hung up and said, "I was right (with a smirk on her face) it is not covered and it never has been so you are responsible." I just said, "OK" because I had been in these conversations before and wasn't going to waste my time with someone who had no authority anyway. I went to pay my $5 office visit co-pay but she did not have change for a $20 bill so she told me to just pay it when I have the surgery. However they sent me a bill the next week anyway with a handwritten note reminding me I forgot to pay my co-pay at the time of the visit when it was required. I sent a $5 check with a note of my own.

The next morning I called the insurance company myself and explained the situation. Turns out the two-tooth minimum is a long standing policy that still makes no sense to me. Do they feel you should be able to withstand the pain of one tooth but not two? Anyway I knew there are always exceptions and I asked if a review could be done. The associate with the insurance company was very helpful and understanding (being nice, explaining the situation and being knowledgeable about my policy along with the process makes a big difference) as she said, "That was just what I was going to suggest." So I had the surgeon's office fax over the proposed bill and the written information regarding my health condition and medications (again I always provide this to a new medical professional to ensure they have all of my current information) to the insurance company then followed-up to ensure it was received. Then I waited.

I followed-up that next Thursday and left a voice message, then on Friday I received a return call from the insurance company. After reviewing my case it was agreed that the IV sedation should be covered at 80%, therefore the allowed amount was now $219 and the coverage was $186.15 while I paid only $32.85. However, the hydrocortisone was not going to be covered and I would be responsible for the $75 cost. A Pre-Authorization Explanation Of Benefits would be sent out to the surgeon's office and myself that day. Overall I was happy and on Monday I paid my new cost of $125 as opposed to the original $365. The surgery went perfectly, I started feeling better and it was a successful experience...Or so I thought.

In a few weeks I received a bill from the surgeon's office for $186.15 and a handwritten note requesting I pay this amount in a timely manner. I replied with a letter stating my insurance company covered this cost and they received a Pre-Authorization Explanation Of Benefits explaining this (how else would they have known not to charge me at the time of service?) and I included a copy of mine just in case they lost theirs. I also had just moved so I gave them my new address and phone number if they had any questions. Again, I thought that was the end of it, but was wrong.

Well, in another few weeks I received another bill with a stronger-worded handwritten note, this time telling me to send in my payment within seven days or else other action would be taken. It was obvious they had not done anything with my reply; in fact the bill had been forwarded from my old address, which proved my point. I knew what the problem was so I called the insurance company myself, told them the situation then asked what type of claim form had been sent in? Sure enough, the surgeon's office had sent in what's called an "In-For-Pay" claim form as opposed to a "Pre-Authorization" claim form, which should have been sent in based on the Pre-Authorization Explanation Of Benefits they had received. The insurance associate made the adjustment to the claim right then so a payment would be sent to the surgeon's office and told me to please inform the surgeon's office they do not need to do anything because we have done their job and taken care of it for them.

So I replied with another letter (after I left a message on their voice mail that was never returned) explaining the situation and we had taken care of it for them so please don't do anything, along with copying the surgeon with the same letter as well. As previously stated, it's good to let the actual doctor know when these types of situations occur because most times they don't keep up with the billing but should know what kind of hassles their patients receive from their staff so they can address them, if they prefer. In a few days I received another Explanation Of Benefits stating the $186.15 had been paid and, of course, never heard from the surgeon's office again.

This is a perfect example of not taking the first quote you receive when you feel it is not right and never pay a bill you know is not right just because there are intimidating remarks written on it. Attempted intimidation doesn't make a wrong situation right but is a more common practice than you might think once you start questioning cost or anything for that matter. I've heard many examples where doctors and others make very defensive and over the line remarks when they are questioned, especially when they don't have an answer. But once again it's your money and rightful benefits at stake here so it's your responsibility to fol-low-up and continue to question until you understand; no matter how frustrat-ing it might be.

My last example is in regard to generic verse brand name drug cost. Most insurance policies today that have drug coverage usually tell you of the three-tier pricing structure. In my case it's $10 for generic, $15 for brand and $30 for drugs on the non-preferred list. I'm not sure how a drug stays off this "non-preferred" list although I'm sure a lot of politics and who knows what else determines who's who. It seems that the majority of my medications this year are on the list but since they work for me I pay the extra money.

While I was employed with EDS in 2002 I went to have my DDAVP spray (for my diabetes insipidus) refilled in January and when I went to pick it up the price was $95 instead of the usual $15. Now DDAVP is an expensive drug to begin with and I always have my Endocrinologist write my prescription as DAW (Dispense As Written), which means I get the brand name. When my Pharmacist followed-up as to why it was so high they were told that since a generic was available I had to use that or else pay a calculation that read "actual brand cost minus actual generic cost plus co-pay", which in this case came to $95 per month instead of $15 per month. Now for me that has a major impact on my budget each month!

So I had my Endocrinologist call in a new prescription for the generic, which I got for $10 while in the meantime I searched through all of the paperwork and documentation I had regarding my new policy to find this calculation or even a mention of it, but was unsuccessful. I even asked my co-workers if they had any documentation mentioning the calculation and none did. But the real problem was with the generic drug itself.

You know how you always hear that there's no difference between the brand and generic drugs except that you pay extra for the brand name because they all have the same active ingredient. Although in some cases this may be true, I've never really believed it. For example in other products there is an obvious taste difference between a Pepsi (brand) and a store brand cola (generic) not to mention the time it takes for the generic cola to go flat once it's opened, even though they have the "same" ingredients. There is also a difference between a pair of Nike running shoes (brand) and a pair of discount store running shoes (generic) although they are made of the "same" ingredients. Not only do the Nike's feel better on your feet but also they last longer (Adidas and Rockport are just as good, just so I plug the other main brand of shoes I wear). My point is there has to be a difference in something and DDAVP is a perfect example.

The brand name DDAVP does not have to be kept in the refrigerator while the generic brand must be refrigerated. So everything else aside there has to be something different between the two for this obvious difference in how you maintain them. It is also clear as day when DDAVP works or doesn't and for me the generic did not work but a very short period of time. This was especially hard at night as now I was getting up to urinate about every couple of hours or so (almost as I was before my diagnosis) and was taking up to four sprays a day as opposed to the normal two a day at that time in my life. This was not good because you have to be careful with DDAVP because if you retain too much water in your body that's as serious as not being able to retain water. But what was I to do since I couldn't afford the extra $85 per month without giving up another necessity?

I tried the generic for a month or so hoping my body would adjust but with no such luck. It was now around the first of February and I knew I had to do something. I got a refill of the generic then started the appeal process by contacting my HMO and submitting documentation from my doctor. In the meantime I still searched for documentation that mentioned this calculation. Neither my HMO (they only got a response from the pharmacy division stating this was the calculation) nor any of my co-workers with the same coverage could find anything in writing mentioning this calculation, just the three-tier price structure.

Around the first of March (exactly 34 days after I filed my appeal) I received a letter stating I had won my appeal. Excited that I was going to be able to get a good night's sleep again I called in my refill of the brand name, but when I got there it was still $95. Come to find out my appeal victory was so I could override the requirement of only getting a month's supply so therefore I could get a refill of the expensive brand name. This was totally useless! Not only because of the fact that wasn't what the appeal requested and I have no idea based on the information in the appeal and my doctor's documentation how they came to this assumption, but simply for the fact it took 34 days for the decision and I could have gotten a refill after 28 days without the appeal…It made no sense!

My HMO told me there was nothing they could do and I had two choices. First, I needed to go to my employer since they were the ones who determine what benefits I had. Second, I could file an appeal with the State Insurance Commission although I'm not sure how they could override my claim but that was what I was told. So for the entire month of March my employer researched my problem as they attempted to find this calculation since it was nowhere in any of my documentation, or as it turned out, theirs either.

Finally, during the last week of March my employer came back and told me they had found the calculation and the reason I did not have it was because in Michigan (I'm not sure if this is Federal and it was the year 2002) the insurance company did not have to provide the subscriber with all of the fine print of your policy until after 120 days from the time the policy started…Legally! So basically they had four months before they had to tell me what I had committed to based on information/documentation I was provided, and let's not forget I can't change policies until my next enrollment, which was not until January 2003.

Although nothing surprises me anymore regarding the health care industry, this was just difficult for me to swallow. Think about this for a second. Is there any other product you would purchase (I did have other choices and I'm partially paying for my coverage) without knowing exactly what you are purchasing and the effect it will have on you and your family's life then not being able to change or return the product when, after the fact, you find it creates major problems for you and just doesn't work for you…Legally? That answer is obvious! To put this in perspective, what if you bought a television set, then when you get home the television will not pick up cable and you weren't told of this. Then you go back to the store and the store then gives you the fine print that states the television is not made for cable. Even though you took the time to check every piece of documentation available beforehand, because this was an important requirement for you, you are not able to return or exchange the television set. You're stuck with a product that doesn't give you what you need and it was no fault of yours because you did all the research with what was available to you before you bought the television to ensure you could have cable. This would be unheard of. So why can HMOs get away with it?

My next step was going to be to write the State Insurance Commission, however on April 3ʳᵈ I was part of a workforce reduction, therefore my wife picked up coverage with her employer. Now even though her coverage was with the same HMO, her policy allowed me to receive the brand DDAVP at my $15 co-pay. This shows how it's actually your employer who determines your coverage, not the insurance company. So I figured it was a non-issue now so I left it alone as the next week I finally received my fine print that mentioned the calculation. Again life was good.

When it was time to enroll in our 2003 benefits, again the cost of my DDAVP was a top priority. Since my wife worked in Human Resources we were able to see the "Non-Preferred List" and other information. All signs pointed to the fact I would still be able to get the brand name DDAVP at my brand co-pay of $15. I got my first refill in January 2003 and sure enough it was $15, no problem.

However, when I got my next refill the first of March my cost was $101. "Here we go again!" I thought to myself when my Pharmacist called me on my cellular phone just as I was on my way to pick up my prescription. Since we both had already been through this before we were at least aware of the issue. A side note...Your Pharmacist can be a valuable asset to both your health and pocketbook so please try to establish a good relationship between the two of you. My Pharmacist had already called my insurance company and they told him that there had been a change in their pricing policy on February 24, 2003 and now the same calculation we had trouble with in 2002 was in effect once again.

But wait...This seems like another example of unfairness when it comes to the rules the insurance company must follow and the rules the subscriber or patient must follow. How is it fair and legal for the insurance company to change their pricing and/or benefit coverage during the covered year but the subscriber or patient can't change or cancel the policy until the end of the covered year? As I stated previously, what other product has to follow these rules where they can change what you purchased and there isn't anything you can do about it? Would you pay an additional $100 for that television set two months later that we described earlier and you still can't get cable but now your local channels don't come in either? Of course not! That situation would never even come up because it's ridiculous. So why can the insurance industry get away with it?

I called my insurance company to verify what my Pharmacist told me and he was correct. In fact, the clerk told me that benefits and pricing are changed all the time. "That's just how it works" the lady on the other end of the phone stated, "Nothing you can do about it". I told her that what I wanted was the address of whom I needed to write an appeal letter to. There was no need in wasting my time with her; after all I had learned that lesson in 2002. She gave me the address and I went to my computer and started documenting the entire situation, giving detailed information regarding what I was appealing and detailed reasons as to why the generic DDAVP didn't work and that there had to be a difference since one required refrigeration and the other didn't...Common sense told you that something had to be different. This time there was no way they could not understand what I was appealing!

I also copied my Endocrinologist because you always need to keep your doctor in the loop. No one likes to be blindsided, especially a doctor who is going to help you. Honesty and good communication between patient and doctor is key to a successful relationship and successful results. I've got to drive that point home!

A few days later I received a letter from my insurance company letting me know they had received my appeal and they were requesting permission to pull my medical records to research my use of DDAVP, which I must return within three business days. They said within 15 days I would have a decision or reply if more time was needed, along with providing me a copy of their Grievance Policy. I granted them permission and returned the form the next day.

In about two weeks I received another letter from the insurance company. After three paragraphs telling me the details of my policy and how the drug pricing works they finally stated, "*After a thorough evaluation, you will be pleased to know that we have decided to approve your request. Therefore, an authorization, which is valid for prescription coverage of the brand DDAVP for one (1) year, has been placed in the pricing system. However, because the brand DDAVP is considered a "non-formulary, non-preferred" product, the highest tier copayment fee of $30.00 will apply.*"

I actually won my appeal with one letter and very little effort, compared to other situations that is! Hey it might not have been at $15 but $30 was a whole lot better than $101 per month. I was satisfied although I still think it is unfair that the insurance company (or corporation) can change their coverage but the subscriber or patient can't.

Then a few months later my prescription for DDAVP doubled from two sprays a day to four sprays a day due to complications with my diabetes insipidus. What this meant was that now I required an additional bottle per month. Each bottle gives you approximately 50 sprays so with two sprays a day I use 60 sprays per month, which constitutes two bottles per month. Now with four sprays a day I would use 120 sprays per month constituting three bottles per month. When I went to get the new prescription we were back to over $100. As we researched we found the appeal was only for the two bottles per month, so therefore I had to go through the appeal process again in order to get the three bottles. So I did and within the same timeframe as previous I won the appeal, only this time for some reason they made the generic $30 as well. Don't know why nor did I care since I was going to use the brand drug. So again life was good in regard to my DDAVP.

The bottom line to these examples is that you must advocate for yourself because if you don't take control of your own situation then no one else will and you will lose out on what you are entitled to. If you can't understand your policy or don't understand what you need to do then ask your caregiver or anyone and everyone you know until someone helps you understand. Do not be embarrassed or afraid to ask as many times as it takes to understand. You have everything at stake here so do what you have to do.

I can proudly say that I've won every dispute and appeal I've ever fought to date regarding my insurance policy billing me incorrectly (as most of the time it was not the insurance company but the doctor's office who submitted the wrong codes or forms). Some have taken a lot of determination, follow-up, persistence, frustration and time, but it was well worth the effort to not only save myself money I shouldn't be spending in the first place, but more importantly, just the satisfaction that I was correct in the fact I received the benefit I was entitled to and paid for. If I hadn't taken the steps to advocate for myself then I never would have received that benefit. Principle for me is the most important personal factor in anything!

Now you might ask, "Why should I take all the time and effort for a few bucks?" Well let me tell you a few reasons why. First of all, because you are entitled to the benefit or service and I'm sure you are paying for the benefit as well. Would you go into another business, say a grocery store and pay for a steak then tell the store to go ahead and keep the steak along with your money because it was on sale anyway and you didn't feel like carrying it to your car, after all it was only $6.95? Of course not! In fact if you forgot it on the checkout stand you would probably drive back several miles in rush hour traffic to pick it up saying all along, "It's mine, I paid for it!" So why would you pay for an insurance benefit then say, "That's okay, I don't feel like making a call or following up myself, keep my money?"

Secondly, the insurance company and doctor make enough on you as it is without you just giving them a double dose of your money. Think about the fact that the $10 they charged you incorrectly, if they charged 200,000 patients that cost and only half of them (100,000 patients) challenged it and the other half (100,000 patients) just paid it, then someone just made $1,000,000…Unjustly. At least do it for the principle of fair business ethics if nothing else!

I want to give you something else to think about financially. As a chronically ill patient (regardless of the condition), it has a financial impact on your life and your family in a variety of ways. There are the obvious such as medical bills and medications. But think about your situation for a second as I give you an example of mine to show you how things you might not think about cost you money. As someone who suffers from diabetes insipidus I have to urinate more often than the average person, especially when my DDAVP starts to decrease its efficiency but yet it's not time to take another spray. That's just how it is. On average a normal person might urinate once or maybe twice between dinner and time to go to bed then maybe get up twice during the night or morning for a total of say four times. In my case I will urinate at a minimum of five times (<u>minimum</u>) before I go to bed then once before I actually go to bed after I've taken my nightly DDAVP. During the night I will urinate an average of three times before morning for a minimum total of nine times. So you ask, "Asides from the hassle, what's the big deal?" The deal is that I flush my toilet an average of nine times per night compared to you flushing four times, which comes to five more times a night for me. In a 30 day month that's 150 more times! The effect is very apparent when I receive my Water & Sewer bill. If your water and sewer cost is anything like ours in Metro Detroit, you will tell a noticeable increase and that's not counting the extra number of times I urinate during the rest of the day. Then on a lesser but real note, I use additional electricity each night to run my CPAP machine for my sleep apnea, gas for multiple trips to the doctor or pharmacy, and so on. So you see, you pay for your health condition in ways you might not even realize. Still wonder why that seemingly small wrong charge is a big deal? Why will you take the time to clip coupons or drive to a specific store to save a few bucks but won't do the same for your medical bills, just because you might not understand or feel intimidated?

The last point I want to make is in regard to those Explanation Of Benefits or invoices from your doctor you get in the mail in which you owe no money. Most people just look at the column that states "$0 due by patient", and then disregard the document. Please don't do that! Before you put it away make sure you check the date of service and procedures the bill is for. Then verify that you actually saw the doctor on that date or a procedure was done on you for that specific date. Unfortunately, it's a fact that some doctors and facilities will bill insurance companies and more often Medicare (because of the government bureaucracy it is easier to get away with) for services rendered that were in fact never rendered at all. Since the patient is never charged a co-pay then they very seldom even notice, much less complain. I've personally seen this on several occasions, while working as a Business Analyst and in my personal life.

It is extremely important that you notice these criminal acts, let's call it what it is, and report it immediately. When reporting it make sure you report it directly to the insurance company or Medicare. Why? Because if the doctor's office or medical facility was trying to get one over then they aren't going to fix the problem for you but instead either cover it up or just stop billing you. If they have done it to you then they are doing it to others so the practice will continue. If it was an honest mistake then it will be corrected when the insurance company or Medicare investigates. Now you might ask, "Why bother? It's no money out of my pocket." Well that is where you are wrong…It's money out of all of our pockets. This is just one reason why, if not addressed, the cost will come back on the patient or customer, or in the case of Medicare, the taxpayer. We are all affected! Please, check all of your bills in detail and address any and every thing that you are not 100% sure of. It really does make a difference.

Advocate for yourself at all times! It's my motto all over again…Understand your reality, realize what needs to take place, then deal with it by any means it takes. Not only for your sake but maybe if enough of us fight the system when the system is wrong then others will not have to go through what we did. Having a chronic health condition is expensive and frustrating enough!

In America we have the greatest health care system in the world (although some people, especially with the cost of medications, might pick Canada), the greatest justice system, the greatest political process and the greatest freedom. But that doesn't mean there aren't problems within the process that cause many people to be treated unjustly. That's what we need to address because that small percentage of wrong could be you the next time! I'll bet you'll have a different point of view if that happens, huh?

9

A DOCTOR'S PERSPECTIVE

❖

What The Doctor Says About Sarcoidosis

Okay, up until now, everything you have ever heard from me, either by way of my writings or speaking engagements, has been strictly from a patient's perspective. This is what I do. I speak for the patient, whether it's from my personal experiences or from what other patients have told me. I'm always looking at it from a patient's point of view. I'm one of the voices for the average person who happens to be a patient with sarcoidosis and many other chronic health conditions. Unfortunately, I have a lot of personal experience as a patient who deals with a chronic health condition on a daily basis. Therefore, I try to help others based on what I've experienced. As I said, "This is what I do."

But what the doctor or medical professional has to say is just as important as what the patient has to say. After all, in order for us to be successful, we must be a team. The doctor must listen to the patient and the patient must be honest with the doctor. Honest communication is the only way to build a successful doctor/patient relationship. From honest communication comes respect. Once respect is earned, on both sides, only then can successful results follow.

Now I've been known to be blunt in my writings in regard to my experiences with the medical profession. In my pre-sarcoidosis days most of those experiences weren't very positive. In fact, some of the post-sarcoidosis experiences haven't been much better. But on the other hand, I've also written bluntly about the many positive experiences I've had with many medical professionals from Primary Care Physicians to Endocrinologist to Dental Professionals to Pulmonologist to Sleep Specialist to doctors I've met through my writings and the many none doctors that I've encountered in the medical field. The bottom line is I tell what happened to me and what has happened to other patients as well. Sometimes the truth can be positive and sometimes it can be cold, but the truth is the truth, and we must look at it for what it is, then we must learn from it.

The human body is a very complicated creation and understanding it is even more difficult. I understand this fact, which again is why I stress honest communication. In fact, I always recommend that you write down your symptoms and questions then provide them to your doctor to ensure you don't forget anything. I can't count the number of times I've had doctors thank me for this process or heard them state that they wish all patients would do the same because it makes it easier to understand what they are dealing with in regard to helping their patient.

The main thing a patient asks of their doctor is, "If you don't know what's wrong, please ask for help." There's no shame in not knowing but it's a tragedy when you don't ask for help and it's the patient that feels the tragedy. I mean no disrespect when I write about the negative experiences patients have endured, so please do not take it as such. Instead look at the situation and do what you can to correct it, whether you see yourself or a colleague in the scenario. If instead you blame me for writing the truth then I must say it's probably a good guess you are one of the problems. Like I tell patients and caregivers to look in the mirror, you, as a doctor, must do the same!

When I decided to write this chapter several things came to mind. First, the main intent is to give a doctor complete freedom to say what they want about sarcoidosis. This chapter or the interview portion of the chapter, is strictly from a doctor's perspective, not mine. I want to make that point clear. Secondly, I had several doctors who volunteered their services to me and said they would participate in this book, if needed. Let me publicly say, "Thank you" to those doctors for their support, even those who feel I'm very opinionated, but yet still support me…You know who you are. I really appreciate your honest support.

One of my pet peeves when reading doctors' opinions, listening to them speak or answer questions at a conference, or even seeing them with a patient on some other media, it seems they only talk about their specialty or only their opinion counts. Now I understand that naturally their specialty is what they are most qualified to talk about, but the problem with that is the listeners or readers walk away with the assumption that sarcoidosis only affects the organ of their specialty. For example, if you listen to a Pulmonologist you might assume sarcoidosis only affects the lungs, or if you read an article from a Dermatologist you might think sarcoidosis is only a skin disease. However, we all know sarcoidosis can attack any organ or gland in the body, including the eyes, skin and spine. This fact must always be presented and understood.

So when it came time to decide if I wanted to include this chapter, the answer was "Yes" because I felt strongly a doctor's opinion should be heard. When it came time to decide how I wanted the interview session to go and with whom, that choice, although difficult based on the fact so many qualified and respected doctors had agreed to participate, was one I knew without hesitation. Fortunately, my choice agreed to participate…So enough of my rambling.

I chose to interview Dr. William Sharp, M.D., who practices in Southfield, Michigan, for a couple of reasons. First of all, I have the utmost respect for Dr. Sharp and what he is doing to raise awareness for sarcoidosis, although he isn't one of my personal physicians. I met Dr. Sharp at a support group meeting at Providence Medical Center in Southfield, Michigan, where I was invited to speak around September 2002. The support group was rather small and there was one member who had just been diagnosed with sarcoidosis and this was the first time she had even been around others with the disease, so she was full of questions and the fear of the unknown. In addition, there were several others who were very open about their condition and very talkative, something that is perfect for a support group.

As I started speaking, while still sitting in an informal atmosphere unlike most speaking engagements, the members would interrupt whenever I said something they either could relate to or had questions about, therefore starting a discussion among themselves. After a few more attempts, it became their discussion and I became more of a question answerer than speaker. The leader of the group was going to try and get them to be quiet and listen to me but I motioned for her to let them talk, after all this was a support group meeting as opposed to a conference and the main purpose of a support group meeting is discussion and opening up…So actually this was perfect.

During the meeting Dr. Sharp came in and at that point also started answering questions. I was impressed with how he handled the patients in the group by listening to them and answering their questions until they understood, no matter how many times they asked the same questions, as some of them were pretty emotional. I was also impressed with his down to earth honest approach and his obvious genuine commitment to sarcoidosis awareness. He bought a book from me and even though it was one of those original ones with the editing problems (I later provided him with a Revised Edition), he became a supporter and encouraged others in the medical profession to read it and get an understanding of how the patient feels. He seemed to always put the patient first and didn't try and cover up any wrongs some of them had experienced.

Over the next year or so, our paths crossed several times during speaking engagements, such as the Michigan Sarcoidosis Awareness Day conference and other events. We also have communicated via e-mail and each time I've asked Dr. Sharp if he could be available for anything to promote sarcoidosis awareness, such as television or radio interviews, he has always agreed and together we have been able to give both a patient and doctor's perspective as a result of our appearances.

Secondly, and the primary reason I chose Dr. Sharp, is because his specialty is Internal Medicine, with other specialties being hypertension, diabetes and sarcoidosis. Dr. Sharp is the first doctor you would see with any problems you might have or just for a regular check-up. This is where most patients spend the most time being misdiagnosed before getting to the specialist of the organ affected by sarcoidosis. Therefore, Dr. Sharp has the overall knowledge and experience to detect sarcoidosis at its early stages and get the patient the appropriate treatment in a timely manner, which as we've read, can be critical to the long lasting effect sarcoidosis can have on our lives. He sees the entire picture, not just his own world.

The process was simple. I submitted questions to Dr. Sharp and he answered them in his own words. When he returned the interview, I put them in the chapter as he wrote them. The answers are his, not altered by me…A doctor's perspective.

The Interview…

(Gilbert Barr Jr.)…Dr. Sharp, how would you best describe sarcoidosis in terms a layperson could understand?
(Dr. Sharp)…Sarcoidosis is a multi-system illness, which varies in severity and involvement with each patient. Sarcoidosis can involve the lungs, lymph nodes, liver, eyes, brain, kidney, bones, skin, heart, nasopharynx and even the genital organs. Any or all of these organs can be involved minimally, greatly and simultaneously. This disorder can be silent or severely disabling or even fatal. Sarcoidosis may be discovered on a routine chest X-Ray without any symptoms, or as a part of an ophthalmologic evaluation, or with the appearance of a characteristic skin lesion with absolutely no symptoms. On the other hand, it may be progressively disabling to the point of respiratory failure.

Sarcoidosis will involve the lungs more frequently than any other organ. As stated above, the lung involvement can occur in a minority of patients without any symptoms at all. Sarcoidosis frequently can give rise to a cough, wheeze and shortness of breath. Sarcoidosis can lead to asthma, respiratory failure, right heart failure and even heart block. This illness has been associated with the direct destruction of lung tissue, which can lead to the formation of fungus balls within the lung.

Sarcoidosis frequently will cause joint pain and stiffness. It may also cause uveitis, which is an inflammatory condition of the eye, which may affect ones' vision. Sarcoidosis may affect the liver with or without causing jaundice, a yellow skin discoloration. This illness can cause kidney stones and it may also cause uncontrolled frequent urination due to involvement of a portion of our brain, which regulates our water balance. When sarcoidosis involves the skin, the changes can range from a purple flatten spot to severe dystrophic changes, which may alter the appearance of the nose and face.

(Gilbert Barr Jr.)…When you see a patient for a specific problem or maybe for just a regular check-up, what are some symptoms or things you look for that trigger you to test the patient for sarcoidosis?

(Dr. Sharp)…Shortness of breath, frequent non-productive cough and or wheezing are probably the three most common symptoms that may trigger my investigation for sarcoidosis. Weight loss, excess fatigue, fever of obscure origin, changes in vision and the appearance of the characteristic dermal plaques or lupus pernio. I frequently get referrals from local Ophthalmologists for evaluation of uveitis to investigate for the presence of sarcoidosis. I have also been consulted to evaluate the origin of kidney stones in various patients, only later to learn that the patient has sarcoidosis.

(Gilbert Barr Jr.)…I know the answer to this question can vary based on specific cases, but in general, how do you go about testing a patient you suspect has sarcoidosis?

(Dr. Sharp)…The chest X-Ray is invaluable in the evaluation of sarcoidosis because there are several abnormalities that may lead one to the diagnosis, such as the appearance of lymph node enlargement and/or extensive scarring. The gold standard is tissue obtained by biopsy. There is no test that supercedes the pathologic diagnosis in sarcoidosis. The angiotensin converting enzyme (ACE) is a blood test that is frequently, but not always positive in this illness. Serum lysozyme may be elevated in a few.

(Gilbert Barr Jr.)…Do you see standard and routine tests being readily available to test for sarcoidosis in the future, say as we now test for high cholesterol, and what needs to happen today, to get to that point?

(Dr. Sharp)…As a clinician and research advocate, one can only hope for a test which is 100% specific and available through blood sampling. Currently, the ACE test is useful but not 100% specific. Tissue diagnosis remains the gold standard.

(Gilbert Barr Jr.)…What would you like to see improve from a research standpoint in regard to sarcoidosis in order to find the cause, better treatment and a cure?
(Dr. Sharp)…Clearly the level of public and professional awareness of this illness is lacking. Sarcoidosis has never received enough PR (Public Relations). This illness is not cancer nor heart disease nor diabetes, but it can disable an individual. I am disappointed in the lack of active research to understand the origin, management and ultimate cure for this illness. For the families of many of the individuals who have this illness, we must increase the number of focus support groups at the local levels. We need more continuing education seminars on sarcoidosis for my professional colleagues so that they may properly treat this illness and inform the public intelligently! There is a great need for additional research funding, along with public and professional awareness of this disease.

(Gilbert Barr Jr.)…How about from an overall awareness standpoint, for both patients and the medical profession?
(Dr. Sharp)…Sarcoidosis is an illness that can have very few symptoms or can be very severe. It is NOT cancer. It can be self-limited or progressively disabling. Be certain that your doctor understands sarcoidosis and cares about your well being. Get more than one opinion when in doubt. This illness, in many instances, can be controlled with the correct therapy. It is also important to be aware of the side effects of therapy and that the appropriate risk benefit analysis occurs before initiating therapy. There are instances where no therapy is required and there are instances where it is an absolute must.

(Gilbert Barr Jr.)…What basic advice do you have for patients with sarcoidosis and those "others" in their lives?
(Dr. Sharp)…It is imperative that the lay community, professional community, including the research community, comes together to facilitate a cure for this problem. There is a great need for additional research funding to accomplish this. It is also very important that the general public become more aware of sarcoidosis and its' consequences. This is why I have devoted a fair amount of time in developing sarcoidosis focus groups, helped to establish a Sarcoidosis Awareness Day,

etc. More help is needed. Write your Congressperson, Legislator, Governor, Benefits Rep, Spiritual Leader, Physician, etc. and make them aware of your concerns about this illness. If we all do a little…A lot will get done.

This interview was conducted in January 2004

FINAL THOUGIITS

As I close, it's now time to remember the last statement I wrote in First Thoughts, which was a Funkadelic song and quote used by George Clinton that goes, "THINK! It Ain't Illegal Yet!" Here are some of my final thoughts...

- This has been a book strictly written from patients' perspectives (except for the previous chapter). Patients can be the best support resource you can have in regard to coping with the daily struggles of living with sarcoidosis or any other chronic health conditions. Not for treatment, for that we need our medical professionals, but for everyday support. Only someone who experiences what you are experiencing firsthand can truly relate to what you feel. Although we are all unique, we are also so similar in so many ways. Listen to their experiences and advice with an open mind...Then you decide and use what's best for you.

- When you read the patient stories in this book and if you look on various sarcoidosis websites that normally have patient stories as well, do you notice that although each case is unique in its own way, there are usually several common elements between them? Things like cold weather kicking off symptoms, sinus problems before the diagnosis, a lot of misdiagnoses, coughing and shortness of breath, muscle/back cramps, skin bumps or rashes, etc. We, as in the scientist, researchers, medical professionals and even patients, must somehow begin to connect the dots. There's no real point to this bullet except to plead for everyone to "THINK!"..."THINK!"...THINK!" Surely someone can come up with the complete picture!

- Often, we as caregivers and parents or even friends, are taken for granted. When you feel you are being taken for granted, especially as a caregiver or parent, remember that in reality that is the ultimate compliment. See, in order to be taken for granted, that means that you have been there and came through each and every time. Why else would the patient or child take you for granted? So be proud if someone takes you for granted because that only means you are taking care of business. Oh, on the flip side, if you are a patient, child or that friend, remember that the person you take for granted is a human being and all human beings like to be thanked every now and then. So make sure you let them know, you know you take them for granted and thank them from the bottom of your heart. Understand how lucky you really are to have them in your life…Not everyone is so fortunate!

- Make sure your caregiver is aware of your personal and medical information, so in time of emergency they can give the information to the appropriate personnel. This information should be carried in the form of a wallet card listing all your vital medical information or either by using a medical alert service, which you wear on a necklace or bracelet…Or better yet do both. Also make sure your caregiver knows where your insurance card is because that will make a major difference in the type of service you receive. Your caregiver will be your lifeline in time of emergency, so make sure they are prepared!

- Everyone deals with his or her health issues differently. As a caregiver or friend this is a fact we must accept and support. As a patient we must understand how we deal with it ourselves so we can eliminate undue stress on ourselves. A perfect example I like to use to bring this point home is grieving. The cause of this process is the same for everyone; someone close to you dies. However, how each individual handles this process is quite different. Some need to talk to family members or friends and remember the times spent together while others just want to meditate alone in peace. Some need to get right back to work while others need time to sort things out. Some are very emotional while with others it might take years to shed a tear. Whose way is right and whose way is wrong? The answer…There is no right or wrong way. Whatever works for you is your answer.

- Kipy provided some tips (based on her experiences) regarding living with sarcoidosis that I thought were of value and wanted to share. They are: Learn to pace yourself (don't push yourself, it will only make you worse)…Listen to your body (when you feel weak, rest)…Take frequent rest periods (this helps to re-fuel your body)…Try to stay positive (remember to be thankful for the things that you can still do)…Be thankful for your loved ones (even though they may not understand what you are going through, they still love you)!

- In addition, Kipy provided more useful advice for anyone who wants to start his or her own chat room or message board. Ask yourself if you are up to the commitment it takes to organize and moderate a group…If you feel you will need help then try to find someone who can share the responsibility of being there each week…Believe in yourself and know that others will need you to be there for them…Believe in what you are doing…Ask God to lead you and trust in Him completely, for God makes all things possible!

- Never be afraid to ask any question as many times as you need to regarding something you are feeling health wise, getting an understanding of your insurance policies, understanding how to take your medications, side effects of those medications, costs you are going to occur for medications or procedures, your diet or for that matter anything you do not fully understand. No question is a stupid question…Period. The only DUMB question is the one that you were afraid to ask! Never be afraid to ask a question to anyone, because you are not stupid for asking but instead stupid for not asking because not knowing could cost you your life!

- Whenever you go to one of your physicians, bring two printed copies of all of your symptoms along with any questions. Keep a copy for yourself to write the responses on and give the other one to the health administrator. If they don't have an immediate answer to your issues, you will remember to bring it up the next visit and hopefully can get a response.

- Understand all of your insurance policies! You must understand what you are entitled to from a benefit perspective and make sure your caregiver is aware of your coverage and where your written documentation is located in case of an emergency. Know if a benefit is covered beforehand by asking, not assuming, because it will be easier to deal with beforehand than after the fact. Question any bill or denial you feel is not correct by following up yourself with the medical professional and/or insurance company, then do whatever it takes to get what you are entitled to. Don't let your frustration cause you to quit because I guarantee you that you will get frustrated many times over. Keep advocating for yourself to the end. It's your money and health that's at stake, no one else's…Bottom line!

- When filing for Social Security benefits here are a few tips I would recommend: Get a good attorney you trust from the start…Get an understanding of the process…Talk honestly to your doctors beforehand because their input will be critical…Document everything…Keep everyone in the loop with all communications…Be patient…And last, but not least, do what you must to survive! Hopefully we will soon have legislation for sarcoidosis that will make the process easier and those who need help can receive it without further causing hardships to their lives.

- Tips from others who have been through the Social Security process: Be sure to obtain a copy of ALL of your test results—these can be very important in a final Social Security disability decision. Look up the Social Security site on the Internet (you can get this link via my website) regarding disability benefits and read everything there is to know about any of your symptoms. For instance, if you have liver involvement, read the specific clauses as to test results that will qualify you for disability benefits. The Social Security Administration and even a good attorney might not know all of the nuances of each side effect.

Some Random Thoughts & Questions...

- Do you think if drug companies didn't advertise so much maybe they wouldn't pass on that cost to the consumer (patients) and our drug costs might go down just a little bit? I just can't understand why prescription drugs cost so much in America and not in other countries when it's the same drug and pharmaceutical company distributing the drug. Don't tell me about the cost of research and getting the drugs FDA approved as the reason, because even the cost for drugs that have been on the market for a long enough time to make the investment monies back are outrageous, especially the ones used by more patients. Tell me about profits for the pharmaceutical companies, their share holders, the insurance companies who by some process (I'm sure money is involved) puts a drug on its preferred or non-preferred list and even some doctors who will only prescribe certain drugs regardless of the choices for other drugs. In findings from separate studies released by the AARP and the consumer group Families USA, brand name prescription drug cost rose three times the rate of inflation in 2003. In fact, it was found that since 2000, the drug prices have risen 27.6%, per the AARP, while inflation has risen 9.3% for the same period. Don't you think it's time we, as patients, start crying foul as loud and often as we can, to anyone who will listen, like our elected officials? Don't you find it strange that the Congress put on such a front by bringing in cots and spending all night to get the Medicare prescription benefit bill passed in late 2003 with a bill so large and containing who knows how many line items that had nothing to do with drug coverage because it was so badly needed for the American people and the government cared so deeply, but yet it will not be fully implemented until 2006…Two years after the election and two years before the next one? We all know it's needed now so why wasn't it implemented immediately or at least within a year? Maybe because it really benefits Corporate America and not the patients, then by the time the patients see what the bill really did for them it's too late to not reelect those who passed the bill and then those same politicians have two more years to cover it up and blame others? Just wait and see! Something has to change because for a lot of us, me included, we must have these medications to survive!

- When is the "No News Is Good News" policy going to stop in regard to informing the patient of their results from medical tests performed on a patient? For all I know, the lab never received my blood work or X-rays, so please inform us one way or the other when our test results come back. Whether it's a general letter telling us everything is okay or a phone number we can call to get the results ourselves, do something! It's hard enough waiting for the results when you think something might be wrong with your health. How are we supposed to know if there is a problem in the lab throwing the results back a few days? We have no way of knowing if the test results are completed unless someone informs us. So if for no other reason, inform us so we can have peace of mind! After all, your mental aspect has a major effect on how you feel, so help us out...It's not that difficult.

• Why won't a pharmacy tell me over the phone which prescriptions by name are ready for my grandmother-in-law but yet they allow me to pick them up without showing any identification? Isn't that a Catch-22 if you ever heard one? If we are going to have privacy protection let's do it right! Maybe a list of who can pick up medications by showing identification. It's time we start implementing policies that make logical sense and work instead of just implementing policies for the sake of implementing policies!

• Why is it that we wait until we can't take it anymore before most of us go to the doctor and especially the dentist? Do we think that if we wait long enough the pain will just go away? We have all done it but isn't it crazy logic?

• Why can't you get into your doctor's appointment by your scheduled time? Surely (except for an emergency situation) there is a doctor somewhere who knows how to make schedules that are kept. In Dearborn, Michigan there's a hospital that guarantees you'll see a doctor in the emergency room within 30 minutes and they do, even on Saturday nights. How can they and others outside the medical profession keep scheduled times, but yet no doctor I've ever seen can? Makes you wonder!

• There's no reason why medical staff, such as office assistants and nurses, can't be kind to patients instead of short and rude, which happens quite often. I realize they are dealing with people who feel bad and they are probably overworked, but that's no reason to not do your job with a positive attitude, as it makes all the difference in a patient's visit. To make my point, someone very close to me had to have chemotherapy at Karmanos Cancer Institute in Detroit. For each session, every single staff person we came in contact with went out of their way to be kind to the patients, even though you could tell they were stretched thin. Not one time in the six visits did I ever see one nurse with any type of negative comment or look, regardless of what they were asked or had to do...Not once! If they can do it under those stressful circumstances, then why can't you? Common courtesy is not just good manners, but in this case, it's part of your job.

- Why is it whenever you get a quote from a doctor regarding a service, a home repair company for home repair, a body shop for body work on your car, or any other similar type of services, there's one price for customers with insurance coverage (higher price) and another for customers without insurance coverage (lower price)? If you're doing the exact same work and using the exact same resources, shouldn't the price be the same regardless of whether you have an insurance claim or not? Then we wonder why insurance is so high!

- Why do companies give better deals to new customers and leave out loyal ones who have been with them for years and are the reason they are still in business? Whether it's a better interest rate on your credit card (new customers get 0% while loyal customers might get 3.9%, if they're lucky) or a better deal on a new cellular phone (new customers get a major discount on most new phones at various locations while loyal customers might get a small discount on limited expensive phones only at the company store). In December 2003 my online provider offered a complete PC for $299.99 for new customers only (I've been with them since 1994), so I couldn't get it as a Christmas gift, even though I would commit to the year contract…And the list could go on. There is always the disclaimer "new customers only" in order to get the good deal. Don't take your loyal customers for granted and treat them as if they do not matter. And then we wonder why there is no loyalty in business today! As I've said, "Wake up to Corporate America's practices before it's too late!"

- Speaking of which…When did a handshake stop meaning anything and your word is no longer stone but instead rubber to be bent to serve your purposes? It seems like no matter what we try to get done, from having a delivery to getting work done on your home, to getting good service in any type of business establishment, to dealing with government elected officials, and I'm not even going to get into the insurance industry, everything becomes a hassle. You will be told anything perceived you might want to hear to satisfy you for the moment, instead of the honest truth. Commitment used to mean something. In my day growing up (I'm talking 1960s–1970s) we believed there were two things no one could take from you. The first was any knowledge you obtained, as knowledge was the key to success, and the second was your word, because when it really comes down to it your word was your bond. Can we, as a society, please try to get back to that principle? Instead of throwback jerseys (that are by the way…Overpriced), let's try throwback ethics (something we can all benefit from)!

Always Remember…

- Be proud of what you look like! It's sad that so many people allow the media and other folks to determine how they should look. Beauty is in the eye of the beholder and more importantly, the eye of the mirror…As in you. If you are thin and feel healthy then great…If you are full figured and feel healthy then great. The only time you should change how you look, except unless you want to, is if your weight (large or small) is causing you to have health problems. Otherwise be yourself, after all if you can't be proud of who you are and love yourself as you are then how can you ever love anyone else? To borrow from a famous quote, "I'd rather you hate me for who I am than love me for who I'm not!"

- I've been asked so many times, that it's worth repeating one more time for those who missed it the first time around…How do you maintain such a positive relationship with your wife with your health situation? Well, we have honest, open communication between us…We are a team and understand that both of us have weaknesses and strengths, the secret being that when one is weak the other is strong…We know how to argue…We trust each other unconditionally…And most importantly—we like each other! It takes hard work but the logic is so simple!

- Children are our future and the elderly are our past. We must care and learn from both because without them there is no us!

- Family is the most important element in life. The strength and closeness of your family is defined by how families come together and support each other during crises, not by how they come together, laugh and eat at family reunions, holidays, barbeques or after the fact. How is your family defined?

- No matter how bad you think you have it…It could always be worse! Never forget that and be thankful for every blessing you have, for nothing is promised you!!!

A Tribute To Kathleen Marie Griffin…

There is one last thing I feel I must include before ending this book and that's a final tribute to a woman who truly displayed a positive attitude towards life, along with doing everything she could to help others and bring much needed awareness to sarcoidosis, a disease she lived with and that eventually had a hand in taking her life…That woman was Kathy Griffin. Kathy was the reason I decided to include other patients stories in this book. The last time we talked I was going to send her a detailed questionnaire after she returned from meeting her father for the first time (a dream of hers) to get detailed information regarding her story. Unfortunately, I never got around to sending the questionnaire. The reason being I knew she wasn't feeling very well and I also knew if I sent the questionnaire she would go all out to complete it for me. That's just how she was. So I held off to give her some time to get herself together health wise. But before I could send it, she passed away.

I thought about how I wanted to write about Kathy, as I still feel that her battle with sarcoidosis from a health standpoint is a valuable story for us all. She suffered with sarcoidosis primarily in her lungs to the point Kathy was on oxygen constantly, along with many, many other issues. But in the same tone, as I've done with all of the patient stories in this book, I didn't want to write her story unless I could get her story from her. Otherwise it would not be fair to the truth of what Kathy dealt with because only the patient can honestly know what that patient experiences…No one else can truly know. Therefore, since I never got the questionnaire to her in time, I decided to write from what I knew about her and her positive outlook on life, which is just as or maybe even more valuable for us all to know than her health issues.

I first met Kathy when she responded to a Press Release I sent to sarcoidosis support groups regarding "*ME & SARCOIDOSIS—A LIFETIME PARTNERSHIP*" in May 2002. She gave me a call and we had a long talk about everything from our personal situations to her efforts to form the only sarcoidosis support group in Northern California, which she called "Hand In Hand", to issues regarding sarcoidosis awareness and how we could improve on getting the word out. She had mentioned my book to her group and several people were interested; in fact she had received several questions regarding my diabetes insipidus condition as well. My wife and I had a trip planned to San Francisco in July 2002 so I planned to get together with Kathy for lunch while I was there. We also started communicating on a regular basis via e-mail.

My first in person meeting with Kathy was special. We met in the lobby of the downtown hotel I was staying at and sat in the lobby cafe, just the two of us. We talked for about two hours on a variety of subjects without ever ordering anything to eat or drink before one of her support group members joined us along with my wife for lunch. Kathy had such a caring and positive personality. She was so easy to talk to as we told each other of our past experiences. On a couple of occasions, as she was describing her battles with doctors and others trying to get people to understand how she felt and to help her, she broke down in tears. It was all I could do to hold back my emotions as well, as I could see the hurt and frustration in her eyes. My heart ached as I listened to her story of going from medical professional to medical professional with no answers, along with the multitude of tests she had to endure, as I could relate all too often. But she would not let you feel sorry for her, as her positive passionate personality would then take over.

Several things stuck out during that two-hour one on one conversation. She was very passionate about starting her support group to not only give sarcoidosis patients and their families a support outlet but to also bring awareness to sarcoidosis in the community. She proudly gave me a Proclamation she had received from the mayor of San Francisco (Willie Lewis Brown, Jr.) declaring August 29, 2001 as Sarcoidosis Awareness Day in San Francisco. In turn I told her about Glenda Fulton and the National Sarcoidosis Society. I was planning on stopping in Chicago during this same trip to meet with Glenda so I told her I would have Glenda give her a call. As it turns out, Kathy became involved with NSS and started a San Francisco chapter. For the rest of her life she had a major impact on fellow sarcoidosis patients with her tireless work with the organization. I can recall on many occasions forwarding her e-mails I would receive from readers asking for support group information in their areas and within a day Kathy would reply with all kinds of positive information for groups in their areas. As I stated earlier, Kathy would always jump into any situation headfirst and not stop until she had succeeded!

There were a couple of personal things I noticed as well while talking with her and in the previous e-mails. For one, she loved to call you "Dear Heart". This was a term she would use in greeting me along with in e-mails as an opening and closing. I think the use of that term is just another example of the way Kathy viewed people…Everyone she knew was dear to her heart as she honestly cared about people. The other thing was in "*ME & SARCOIDOSIS—A LIFETIME PARTNERSHIP*" I have a chapter titled "A Queen Enters My Life" in which I describe how I met my current wife. From that day on she always referred to my wife as "Your Queen". I think she could truly relate to my use of that term in describing my wife and there was just something special about it every time she would write or say it to me. You know…Genuine from the heart!

Another interesting story she told me referred to the hills (although that term doesn't do them justice) throughout San Francisco. I assume most of you have seen pictures or movies of the hills that make up San Francisco (the classic Steve McQueen movie Bullet comes to mind), but if you have never experienced them in person then you can't really relate to how it feels to walk around the city.

Kathy told me when she first moved to the area how going up the hills was so tiring but walking down them actually scared her! She thought she would not be able to stop and end up falling and causing who knows what kind of damage. So when she first started getting around (before her use of oxygen increased) she would literally sit down on her butt and go down the hills by sliding slowly down the sidewalk using her legs and hands, but always staying on her behind. She said she felt kind of embarrassed at first but that was the best way she knew to get where she needed to go.

Now, after we got a chuckle out of that story, I thought about how that defined what Kathy was all about. Regardless of the obstacles before her, whether it was a steep hill to go down or dealing with the daily struggles of sarcoidosis, Kathy found a way to survive and achieve her goals. Her determination and self-motivation should be a classic example to us all. This is just how she went about her life, dealing with whatever came her way in the best possible way she could and always with a positive attitude. But eventually sarcoidosis took its toll.

I was scheduled to give two workshops in March 2003 at a conference in Southern California. Kathy and others from her group were going to attend, so I asked her if she would like to speak briefly at one of the workshops and she agreed. Unfortunately, she was hospitalized during this time and was unable to attend. I later found out that she had been in bad shape. In fact the doctors had predicted she would never leave the hospital alive and even called the family in so they could give Kathy their final farewells, as she was in a coma. But she was not ready to go just yet!

I talked to her for the final time right after that hospital visit and she told me she took it upon herself or "I went on strike" as she put it, to make sure she was taken care of in the manner in which was needed for her to survive. She told me that her family was singing to her while she was in a coma and although she didn't remember any of the songs she was told she was singing with them in a very low voice, although I believe it was actually God singing through Kathy.

Like myself, Kathy believed in advocating for herself, especially when it concerned her health. This is important for us all to do but extremely important for sarcoidosis patients because, unfortunately, at times the understanding of our condition is not always at the level it should be. Therefore, we must take over our own situation and ensure we get the help we need. We really do have the final say but we must understand how to use that power to our advantage…Kathy understood this very well.

During this last conversation she was excited about her upcoming trip to St. Louis to meet her father, but I could just sense a tiring in her voice. I knew her well enough to know she was still not feeling very well but, of course, nothing was going to stop her from living life. A month or so went by and I actually had just written on my calendar to send the questionnaire to her the following week, when after a couple of hours I received a phone call from San Francisco. It was a friend of Kathy's who informed me Kathy had passed away on September 16, 2003 due to complications from sarcoidosis. At the time she was 50 years old with a birthday coming up on December 9th.

Now since I do not know all the medical facts nor was I in San Francisco at the time, I'm not going to speculate on the details of her death. That would not be fair or ethical on my part. By what I was told Kathy was not feeling very well that September morning and decided she should be taken to the emergency room. She passed away soon after!

Kathy was an extraordinary person who did so much positive in her life. I pray that she did not leave us before her time but I'm sure God took her at this time for a reason. Kathy had a strong Faith and I believe in my heart that God has another plan for her. Although it's hard for us who knew her to understand (as the saying goes "She is now in a better place!"), I can only thank God for allowing our paths to cross, as I learned so much from Kathy's positive outlook on life and I miss her e-mails and supportive conversations greatly. I can only imagine how those close to her on a daily basis must feel. She was truly special!

The Challenge…

As I close, I want to issue a challenge to everyone—from medical professionals to researchers to scientists to politicians to the everyday person—who has read this book or heard any of my speaking engagements. Whenever I speak I end every talk the exact same way, by describing the four hopes I have in regard to sarcoidosis and patients. That needs to change! So my challenge I want to throw out is for some great mind or minds or just someone dedicated to the cause, or maybe just some lucky individual to come up with a way to force me to come up with another ending. But until then I'll continue to close in this way.

First, I hope that one day we will determine and agree upon the origin of sarcoidosis, so that we can become proactive in regard to prevention so that future patients will not have to endure what we have, or better yet, will not become a future patient. If nothing else we can at least stop the spreading of the disease if we have an educated idea of how sarcoidosis develops in our bodies and be on the lookout for those circumstances. Prevention is such a valuable advantage to have available to you and future sarcoidosis patients should have that advantage.

Second, I hope that one day we will have standard and routine tests that are run to detect sarcoidosis, with the keywords being "standard and routine" as opposed to biopsies. We, as a people, have the technology and the mind power to accomplish this task, if our efforts and funds are used wisely and without secondary agendas. Future patients should not have to go weeks, months and in cases such as mine, years being misdiagnosed without ever being tested for sarcoidosis, causing life altering secondary conditions to develop just because no one routinely tests for sarcoidosis. This should be unacceptable!

Now let's take it one step further. The tests should not only be administered at our doctor appointments or standard physicals but also be available at free clinics and free health fairs as well. We should have a test for sarcoidosis available just like checking your blood pressure or high cholesterol. It's a fact that in America the number of Americans without health insurance is at a crisis level. Let's face this reality and do something about it. If, as suspected by some in the medical field, a possible environmental agent is a primary cause for sarcoidosis and a source for that agent might be in industrial plants and the pollution they produce, those plants are usually located in poor urban or rural neighborhoods. In most cases (although today the uninsured are in all income brackets) the majorities of the people living in those environments (including the children) have no health care insurance or are on government sponsored plans, which aren't the greatest in the world. Shouldn't those individuals be a primary concern for testing for sarcoidosis? Again we must become proactive before more individuals suffer unjustly what could be prevented! Just because you don't belong to the haves doesn't mean you don't deserve proper health care.

Third, I hope that one day we will have a useful broad legal definition and category for sarcoidosis that is of value so that patients will not be constantly denied Social Security benefits, disability claims, insurance policies and employment opportunities because of a lack of understanding and available accurate information. All sarcoidosis patients don't only have shortness of breath or minor fatigue, a definition I've seen multiple times as the reason for denial when the patients all had different symptoms. Sarcoidosis can affect any organ or gland in the body and because of that fact there can be a wide variation of chronic secondary conditions. The legal definition should clarify that fact and stress to look at the results of sarcoidosis instead of assuming all sarcoidosis cases are the same. It's just not that cut and dry!

We must ensure our lawmakers and politicians understand the importance of sarcoidosis legislation and if they don't then we must use the power of the vote to ensure the next set does. There is too much at stake for sarcoidosis patients and their families to have to deal with constantly being denied for a lack of under-standing…Legally! Our quality of life is just as valuable as anyone else who might need assistance or employment.

Last but certainly not least, I hope that one day we will find and agree upon a cure for sarcoidosis. I don't think this needs any further explanation!

Will someone or group of people please force me to change my ending! Are you up to the challenge?

It's Not The End Of The World…

The human body is such a complicated and interactive machine. I personally think the human body is the greatest creation God ever made. It's truly amazing when you think of all of the things your body does and how it can heal itself or warn you when something is wrong. We need to always keep our options open when we have something medically wrong with us, instead of just looking for the same ole diseases. If your medical professional doesn't want to do that, then find another. Diseases like sarcoidosis shouldn't take months or years to detect. Our society and technology have moved beyond that point. Detection in a timely manner, then the correct treatment for your situation, can allow you to live with any disease. Then by understanding your reality, honestly accepting it and deal-ing with it, will allow you to move on and live a productive life, even with sarcoi-dosis.

My life has changed dramatically since 1986, as I went through the stages of living with sarcoidosis. From the first symptoms and migraine headaches to the years of misdiagnosis to my good fortune of finally finding doctors who helped me. Then the new world of life with sarcoidosis and the multiple chronic health conditions resulting from the organs affected, as I learned how to understand my new reality and deal with it in a positive manner, which still today is a daily adventure. I've gone from a healthy-active-basketball-hard-working individual to someone who must always be aware of the way I'm feeling, remember to take my daily medications, can't do some of the activities I enjoyed the way I once could, if at all, can't plan my future because my future is based on my health on that particular day and can't work a regular job, causing me to feel at times less than a man. But with that said and understood by my family and me…My life is still fulfilling, happy and productive…Even with that no-no word "can't" associated with my life!

I understand my reality and accept it. Therefore I do things within my limita-tions so my health doesn't suffer and I can accomplish activities that make me feel positive, from both a physical and mental standpoint. My family understands my reality because I'm honest with them about how I feel, plus they are with me on a daily basis and they accept it. We are a team and with all teams some members are strong in one area while weak in another. The secret is that at least one of you is strong in every area and shares the load and responsibilities together, without hesitation or complaint. It doesn't matter who does what, as long as everything gets done...True teamwork! We plan our activities based on past situations and realize each day is different. We are not disappointed or expect too much from a single experience and as we like to say, "Just go with the flow." Of course we all would like more of my pre-sarcoidosis life back and frustration is also part of our reality, but our lives have not come to an end because of sarcoidosis. Instead our lives have just changed, which is really what life is anyway...An ever-changing experience. We have grown together and learned from each experience.

I don't want to sugarcoat the difficulties you experience living with sarcoidosis or any other chronic health condition, as that would not be fair or help anyone understand what he or she might face. But I do want to leave you with the message that you can have a very happy and productive life with this disease or any other chronic health condition, for that matter. Take advantage of every opportunity life gives you and always keep your eyes and mind open to the opportunities around you...They are right in front of you. Life is too precious and short not to live it to the fullest of your capabilities. With honesty, understanding, good support and Faith, it's not the end of the world...Just a new beginning! Always Stay Positive!!!

HONESTY...OPEN COMMUNICATION...UNDERSTANDING YOUR
REALITY...TRUST
These are the keys to a fulfilling life and successful relationship on any level
Thanks for your support...Gilbert Barr, Jr.

ACKNOWLEDGMENTS

❖

From The Author

Thanks to those special people who took the time and donated their stories and/ or names of their organizations to this book, specifically...Kipy Barwick...Marguerite Comstock...Ruth Jacobs...Dan Stoddard...Chris Vitale...&...Heather Walker.

Thanks to Carol Dolida, for not only donating your personal story to this book, but also for allowing me to use your proofreading skills once again, even though I know you were feeling bad at times. Sometimes "Thank You" just doesn't convey the true appreciation that a person wants to tell another person...This is one of those times!

Thanks to Dr. William Sharp, M.D. for donating your knowledge and insight from a doctor's perspective. I wish more medical professionals took sarcoidosis as serious as you do!

Thanks to ALL of the support groups, such as Glenda Fulton and The National Sarcoidosis Society, Inc., for your tireless dedication to promoting and supporting sarcoidosis awareness. I wish I could name you all but you know who you are.

Thanks to everyone who has ever e-mailed me. I treasure the communications we shared and as long as I'm able, I'll be available.

To the memory of Barbara Freeman for her support and offering me the opportunity to speak at her support group's Sarcoidosis Awareness Day event in 2002, I'll always remember you as a special person in my life.

To the memory of Kathleen Griffin and to her surviving family...Thank you for allowing me to use Kathy's story in this book. You were truly an Angel On Earth!

To the memory of Jose "Luiggie" Hernandez and all of the positive influences you had on many people, not only with sarcoidosis but their families as well. I'm honored I had the opportunity to know you and the privilege to write your story for this book. You will always be remembered!

Last, but by no means whatsoever least, I thank my soul mate, best friend, personal advisor, personal assistant and partner...My wife, Ma-Shelle. There are not enough words and Lord knows I could never find the right ones anyway, to describe how much you mean to our lives, as we are truly one. So I'll just say..."I Love You & Thank You For Loving Me!"

You can contact Gilbert Barr, Jr. via the website...

WWW.GILBERTBARRJR.COM

Thank You For Your Support

0-595-32114-3

Printed in the United States
27961LVS00005B/322-327